Hair loss

Natural Treatments!!
to get it back

Jose Hernandez

Copyright Page

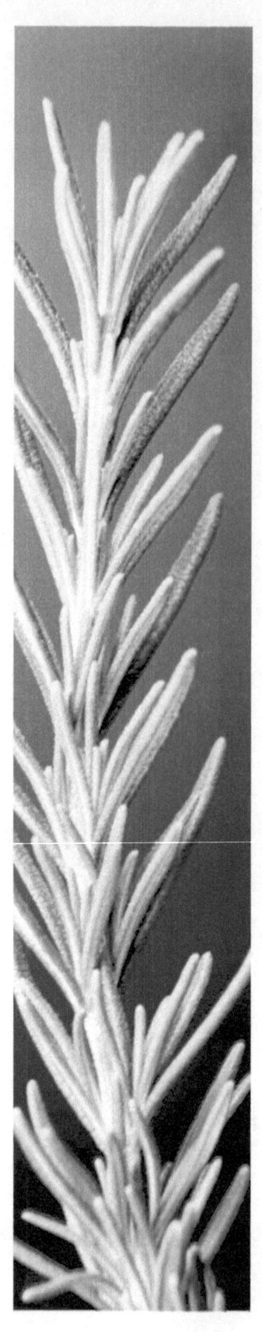

Index

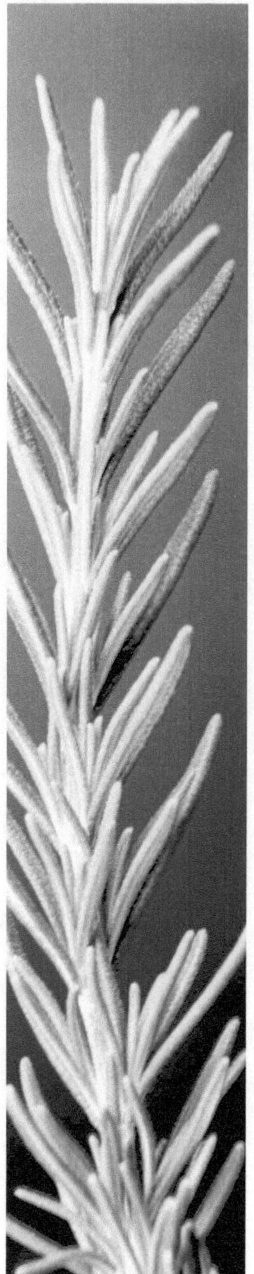

Introduction:

Discover the Natural Solution to Combat Hair Loss.

Welcome to "Hair Loss: Natural Treatments to Recover It", your complete guide to restore the health and vitality of your precious hair naturally and effectively. In a world where hair loss can be a constant concern, it is essential to have proven and safe strategies that address the problem at its root.

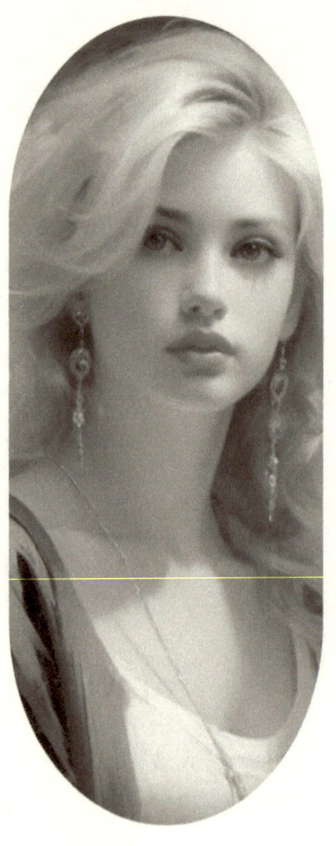

In this introduction, we will explore how to deal with hair loss holistically, using natural treatments backed by ancient wisdom and modern science. You will discover how nature itself offers a wide range of solutions that nourish, strengthen and revitalize your hair, providing you with the necessary tools to regain your confidence and hair beauty.

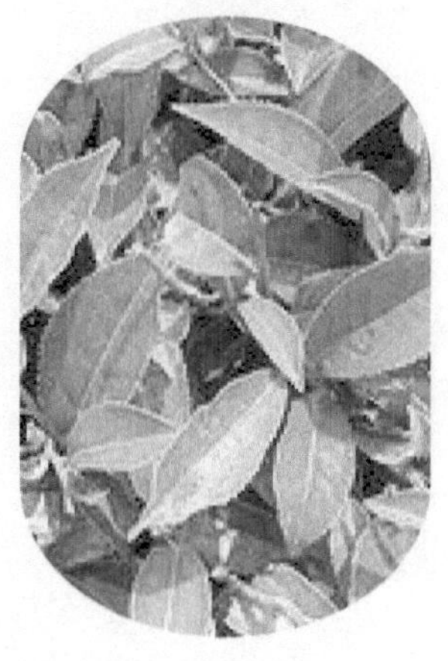

Understanding Hair Loss: Challenges and Natural Solutions

Hair loss is a common problem that can affect people of all ages and genders. From stress and genetics to hormonal imbalances and poor diet, there are a variety of factors that can contribute to this troubling problem. However, with the right approach and the right natural treatments, it is possible to significantly restore hair health.

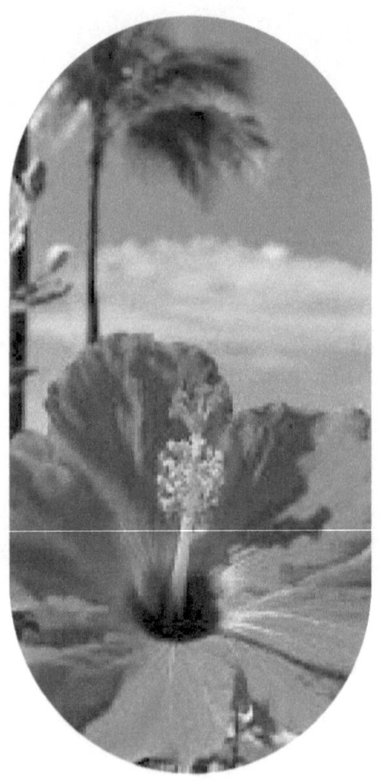

The Power of Nature: Natural Treatments:

for Hair Regeneration.
Nature provides us with an abundance of resources that can help restore and strengthen our hair naturally. From herbs and essential oils to key vitamins and minerals, there are a variety of botanical ingredients that have been shown to be effective in stimulating hair growth, improving scalp circulation, and strengthening hair follicles.

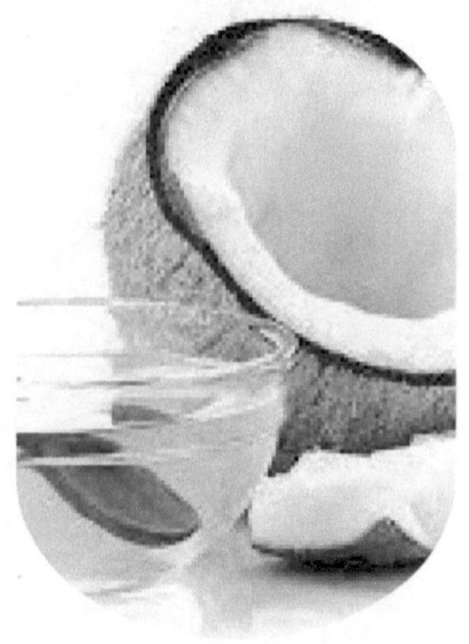

Throughout this book, we will explore a wide range of natural treatments that you can easily incorporate into your daily hair care routine. From homemade masks and scalp massages to nutritional supplements and dietary changes, you'll discover how to harness the power of nature to restore and maintain healthy, lush hair.

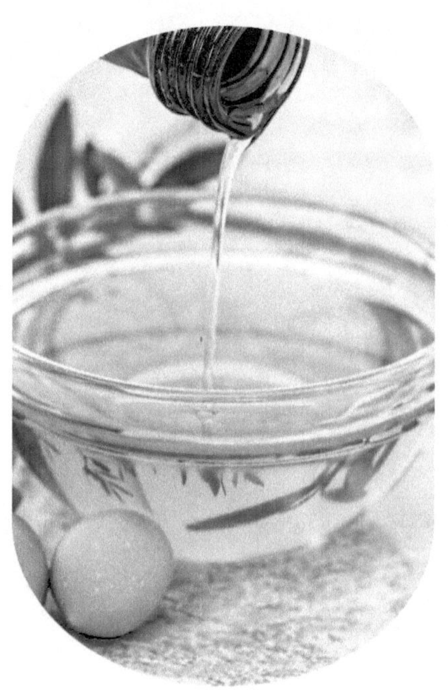

A Step by Step Guide to Hair Recovery

"Hair Loss: Natural Treatments to Recover Hair" is not only an informative resource, but also a practical guide that will take you step by step through the hair restoration process. With clear instructions and expert advice, you will learn how to create your own personalized treatment plan that suits your individual needs and goals.

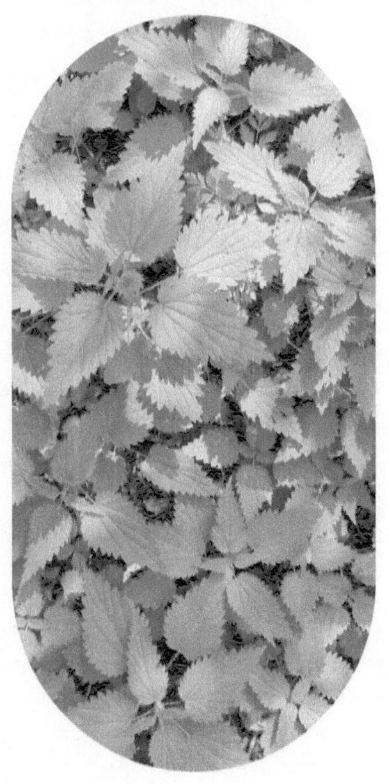

From identifying your hair loss triggers to making changes to your lifestyle and hair care habits, this guide will give you the tools and motivation to start your journey toward stronger, thicker, and healthier hair..

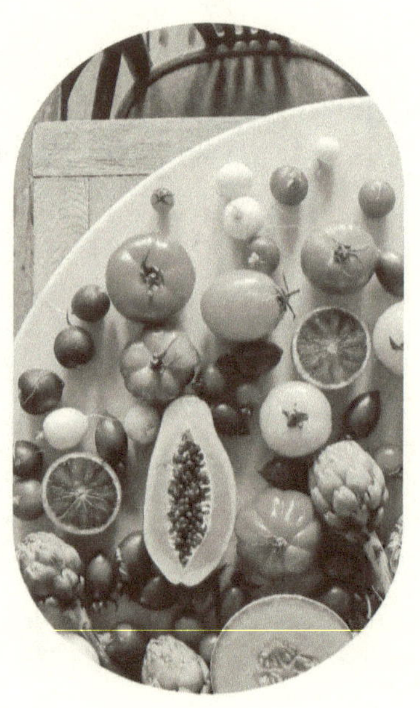

Your Journey to Renewed Hair Starts Here:
Get ready to embark on a transformative journey towards hair recovery. As you explore the pages of "Hair Loss: Natural Treatments for Hair Loss," I invite you to open your mind and heart to the infinite possibilities that nature has to offer. Together, we will take the first steps towards renewed, radiant and full of life hair.

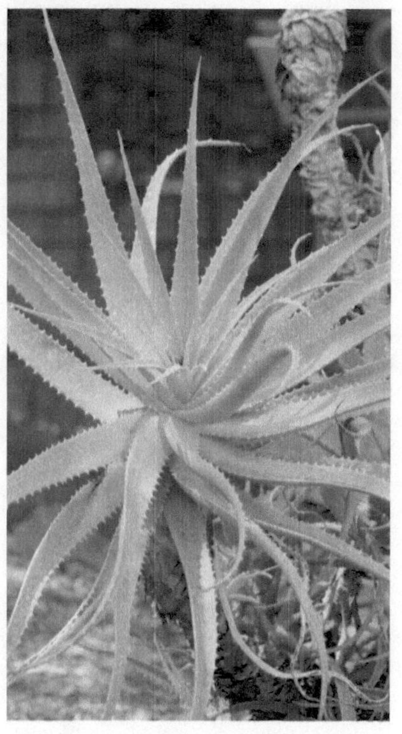

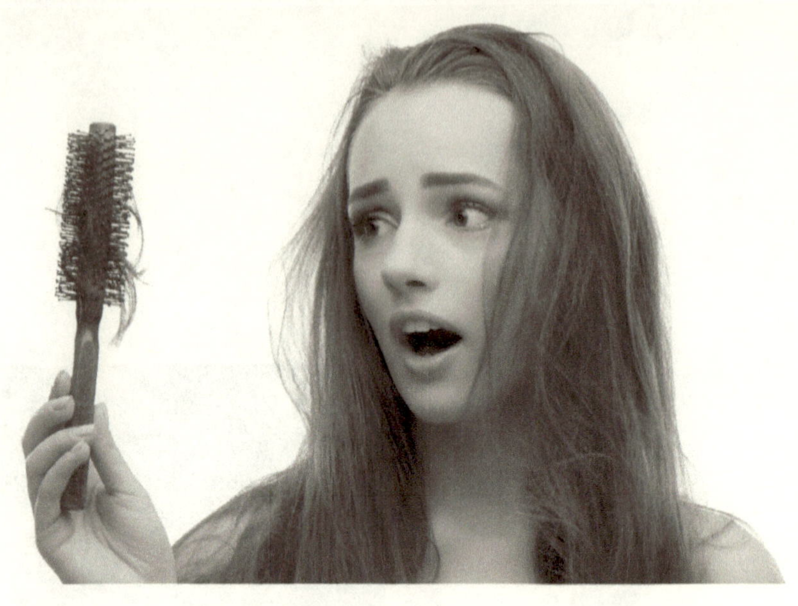

II Causes of hair loss

———————

Hair loss can be a worrying issue for many, but understanding the different causes behind this phenomenon can help us address it more effectively. Here I explain the main causes of hair loss in a pleasant and attractive way:

1. Genetics: The DNA of Hair: Imagine that hair has its own instruction book, and those instructions are written in your genes. If you have a family history of baldness, you may inherit those instructions that may predispose you to hair loss. So, in a way, you can blame your ancestors for that baldness gene!

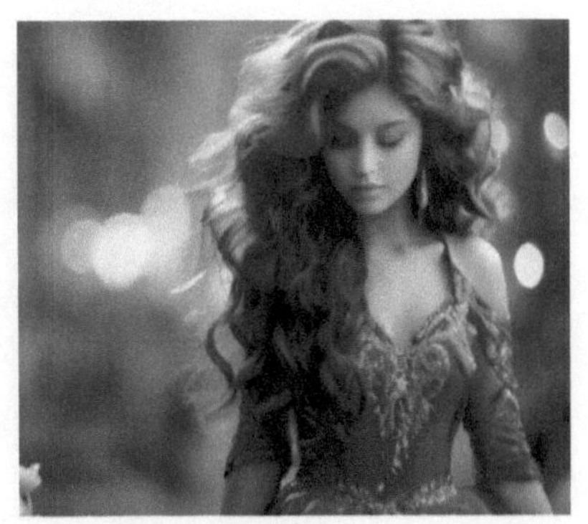

2. Rebel Hormones: The Dance of Hormones: Our body is like a party where hormones dance to the rhythm of music. But sometimes, these hormones can become a little unruly and imbalanced, especially during important times like pregnancy, menopause, or extreme stress situations. When this happens, they can influence the hair growth cycle and cause more hair to enter the resting phase, eventually leading to hair loss.

3. Bad Nutrition: An Out of Tune Diet.

Think of your hair as a plant that needs nutrients to grow strong and healthy. If you are not giving your body the right foods, your hair can suffer the consequences. An unbalanced diet, poor in essential vitamins and minerals, can cause your hair to become brittle and prone to falling out.

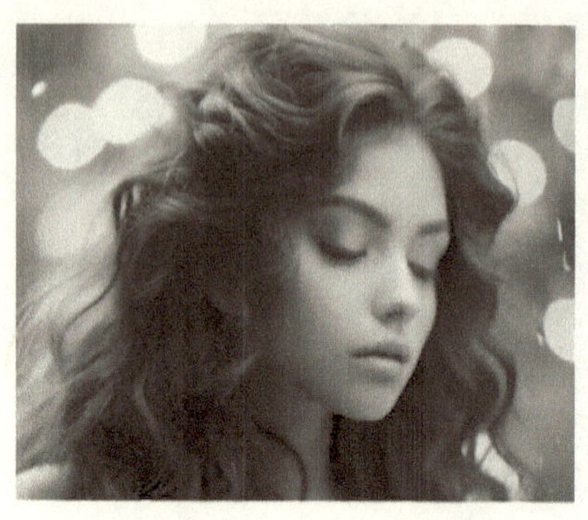

4. Stress: The Weight of the World on Your Shoulders:

We all know what stress is, right? It's like having the weight of the world on your shoulders. Well, that extra weight can also affect your hair. Intense stress can cause hair follicles to go into shock and temporarily stop hair growth, eventually leading to hair loss.

5. Chemicals: The Dark Side of Beauty:

Sometimes the products we use to beautify our hair can turn out to be villains in disguise. Dyes, harsh chemical treatments, and even some shampoos can damage the scalp and weaken hair follicles, causing hair loss.

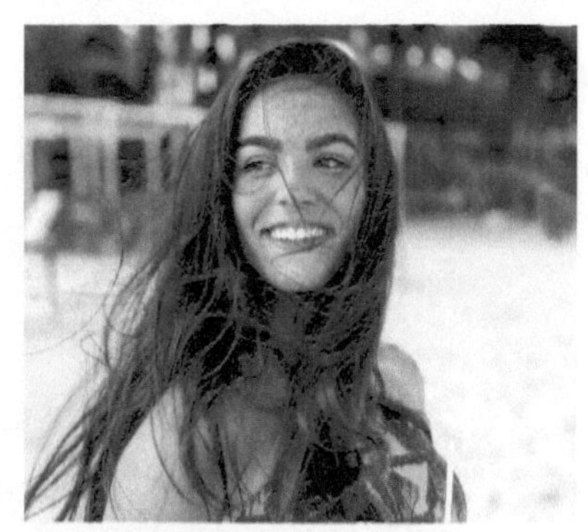

6. Diseases and Medications:

Life's Surprises: Life sometimes surprises us with diseases and medications that can have unexpected side effects, and hair is not immune to them! Some chronic diseases and medications such as chemotherapy can cause hair loss as a side effect.

7. Bad Circulation: Traffic on your Scalp:

Imagine your scalp is a busy city and blood circulation is like traffic bringing nutrients to your hair follicles. If that traffic becomes congested due to poor circulation, hair follicles can be left without the nutrients they need and hair can begin to fall out as a result.

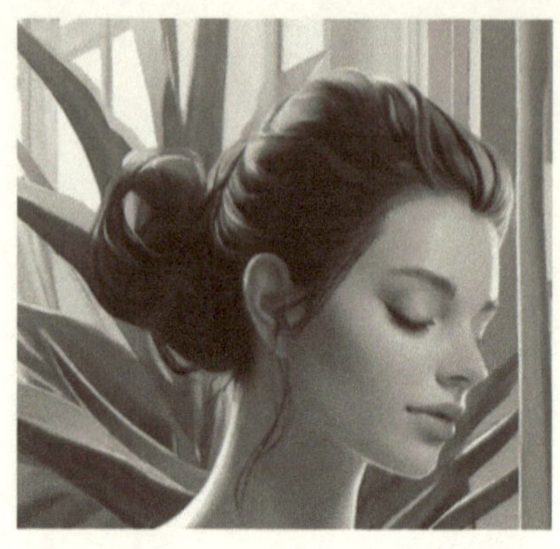

Understanding these causes can help you take steps to care for your hair and keep it healthy and strong. Remember that your hair is a part of you, and while hair loss can be worrying, it can also be an opportunity to explore new ways to care for yourself!

III Natural Treatments

Aloe Vera (Aloe barbadensis) and Coconut Oil (Cocos nucifera) Mask:

Preparation:
·Mix 2 tablespoons of aloe vera gel with 1 tablespoon of coconut oil in a small bowl until you obtain a smooth paste.

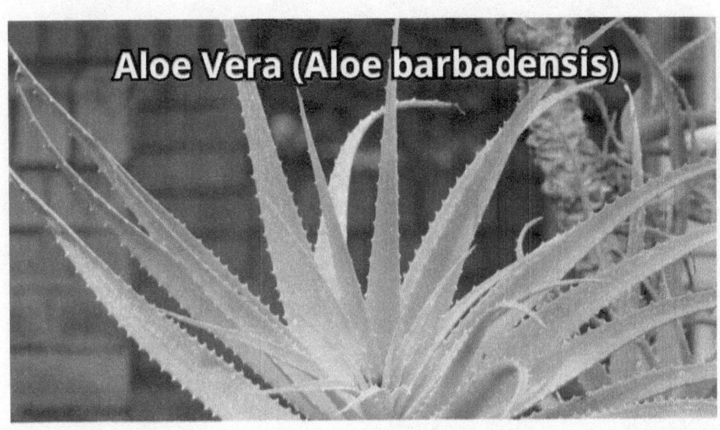

Application:

·Apply the mask to the scalp and massage gently with circular movements.
·Leave it for 30 minutes.
·Rinse with warm water and mild shampoo. Repeat 2-3 times a week.

Infusion of Nettle (Nettle dioica):

Preparation:
·Boil 2 cups of water and add a handful of nettle leaves.
·Let it boil for 10 minutes, then remove from the heat and let it cool.

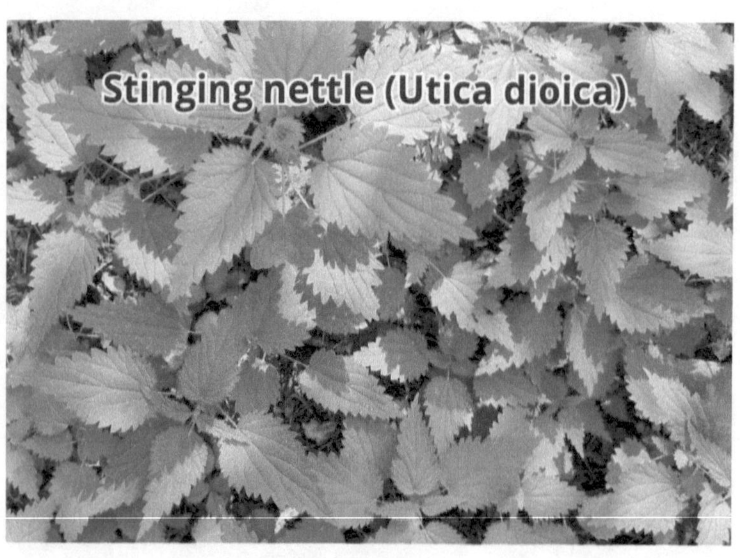

Application:

·Apply the nettle infusion to the clean scalp and massage gently.
·It is not necessary to rinse. Use it as a final rinse after shampooing. You can use it every time you wash your hair.

Rosemary Essential Oil (Salvia rosmarinus):

Preparation:

·Mix 3-5 drops of rosemary essential oil with 1 tablespoon of carrier oil, such as jojoba oil or coconut oil.

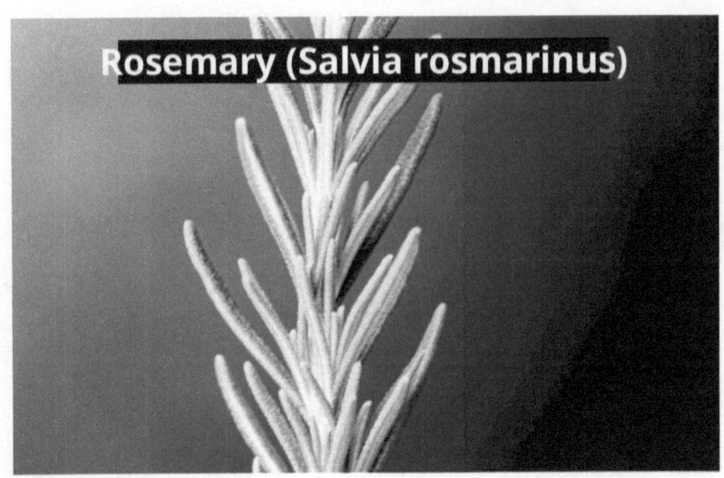

Application:

·Gently massage the oil mixture into your scalp before going to bed.
·Leave it overnight and wash your hair in the morning.
·Repeat 2-3 times a week.

Avocado (Persea americana) and Banana (Musa paradisiaca) mask:

Preparation:

·Mix the pulp of half a ripe avocado with half a banana in a bowl until you obtain a uniform paste.

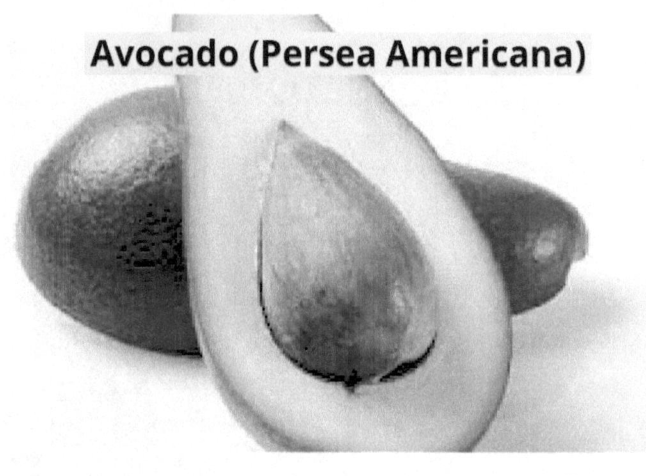

Application:

·Apply the mask to damp hair, making sure to cover the scalp and ends.
·Leave it for 30 minutes and then rinse with warm water and mild shampoo.
·Use this mask once a week.

Apple Cider Vinegar and Rosemary Rinse:

Preparation:

·Add 2 tablespoons of apple cider vinegar and a few sprigs of fresh rosemary to 2 cups of hot water. Let it rest for 30 minutes and then strain.

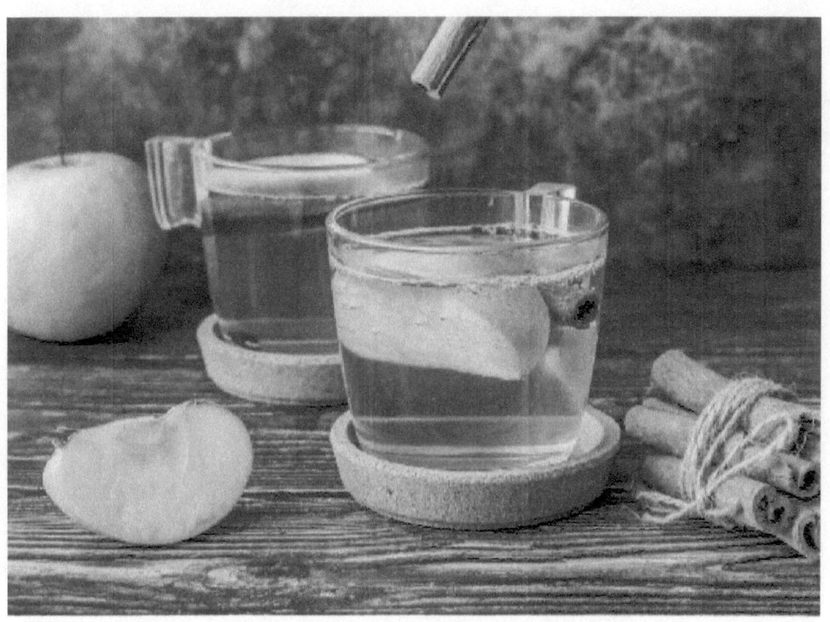

Application:

·After washing your hair with shampoo, pour the apple cider vinegar and rosemary rinse over your hair and scalp.
·Massage gently and leave it on for a few minutes before rinsing with warm water.
·Use it once a week.

Egg and Olive Oil Mask (Olea europaea):

Preparation:

·Beat an egg in a bowl and mix with 2 tablespoons
of olive oil until well combined.

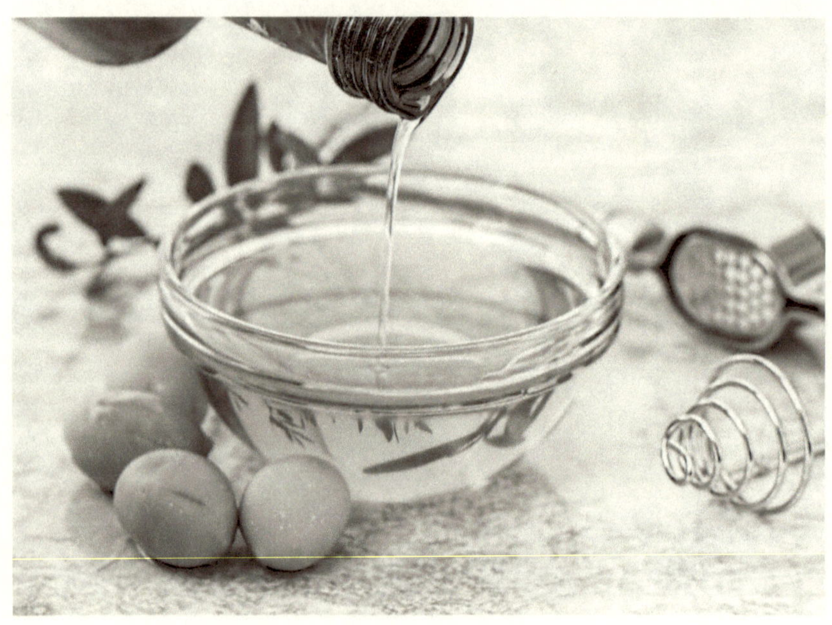

Application:

·Apply the mixture to the scalp and damp hair.
·Cover your hair with a shower cap and leave it on
for 30 minutes.
·Rinse with warm water and mild shampoo. Use it
once a week.

Hibiscus tea (Hibiscus rosa-sinensis):

Preparation:

·Boil 2 cups of water and add 2 tablespoons of dried hibiscus petals.
·Let it rest for 20-30 minutes and then strain.

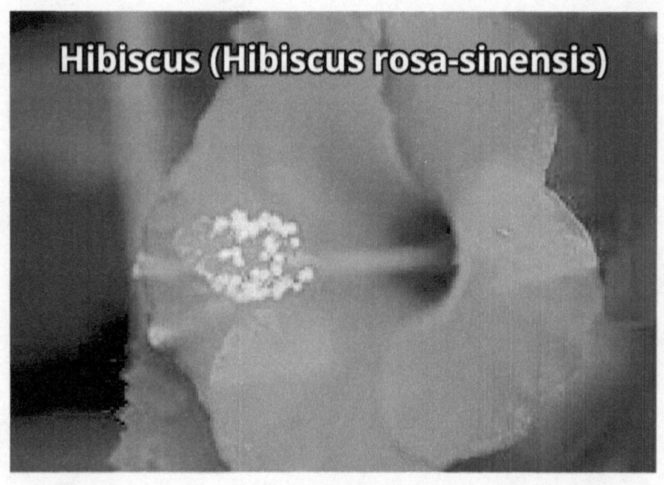

Application:

·Use hibiscus tea as a final rinse after shampoo.
·It is not necessary to rinse. Use it every time you wash your hair.

Rosemary and Nettle Infusion:

Preparation:

·Boil 2 cups of water and add a few sprigs of rosemary and a handful of nettle leaves.
·Let it boil for 15 minutes, then remove from the heat and let it cool.

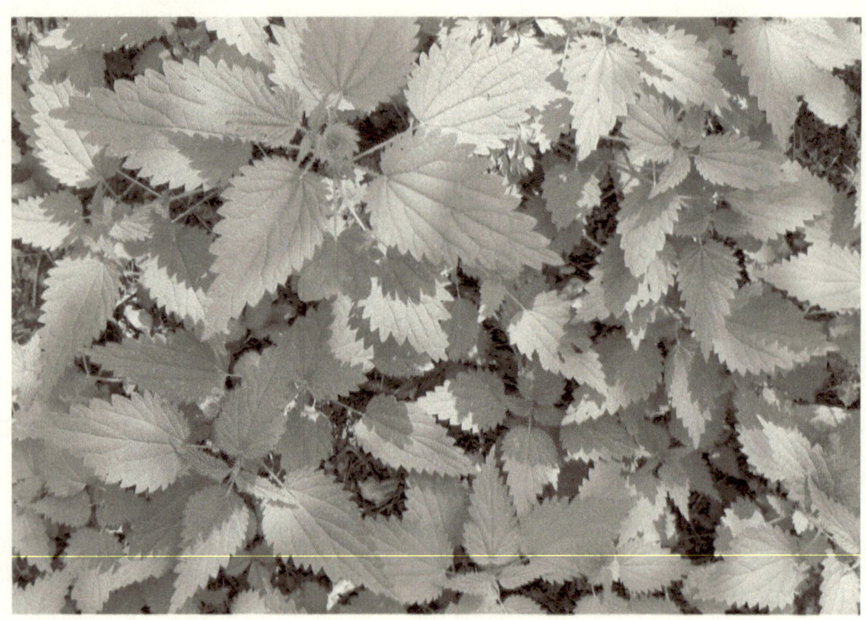

Application:

·Use the infusion as a final rinse after shampooing.
·Massage gently into the scalp and hair.
·It is not necessary to rinse. You can use it every time you wash your hair.

Onion (Allium cepa) and Honey Mask:

Preparation:

Mix 2 tablespoons of onion juice with 1 tablespoon of honey in a bowl.

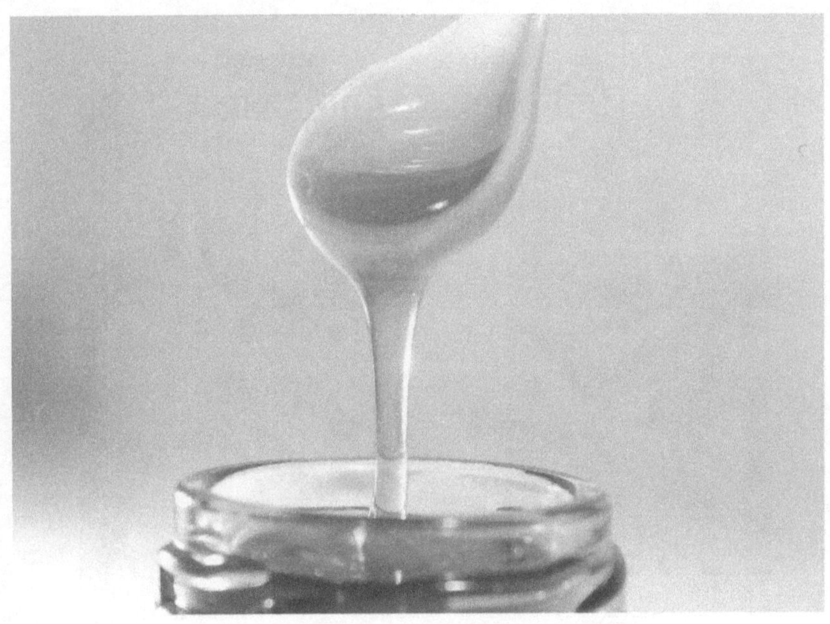

Application:

··Apply the mixture to the scalp and massage gently.
·Leave it for 30-40 minutes and then wash your hair with a mild shampoo.
·Use it once a week.

Jojoba (Simmondsia chinensis) and Lavender (Lavandula angustifolia) oil:

Preparation:

·Mix 3-5 drops of lavender essential oil with 1 tablespoon of jojoba oil.

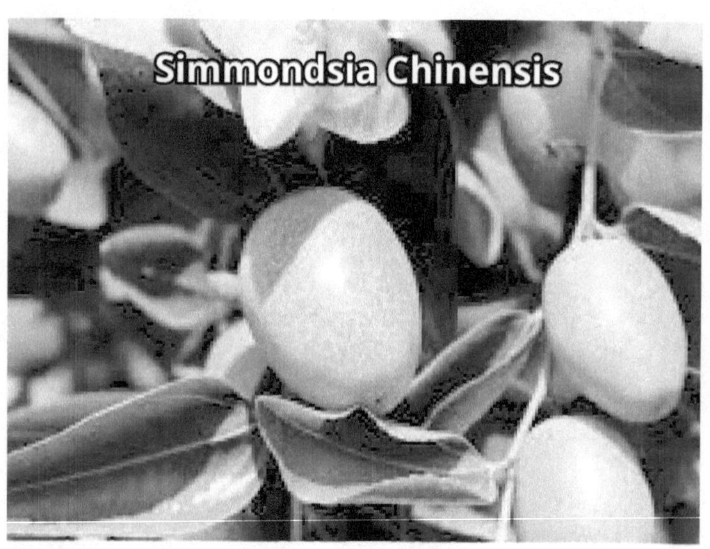

Application:

·Gently massage the oil mixture into your scalp before going to bed.
·Leave it overnight and wash your hair in the morning.
·Repeat 2-3 times a week.

Yogurt and Honey Mask:

Preparation:

Mix 1/2 cup of plain yogurt with 1 tablespoon of honey in a bowl until smooth.

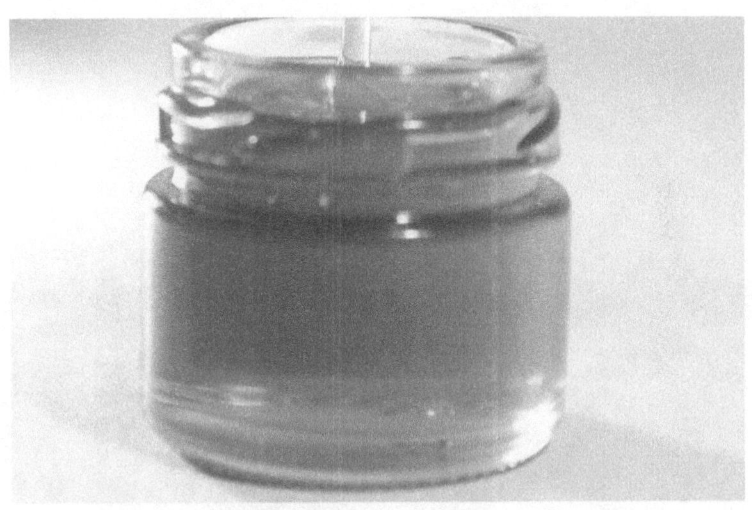

Application:

·Apply the mask to the scalp and hair, making sure to cover all areas.
.Leave it for 30 minutes and then rinse with warm water and mild shampoo.
.Use this mask once a week to strengthen hair and reduce hair loss.

Green Tea Rinse (Camellia sinensis):

Preparation:

Brew a cup of green tea and let it cool to room temperature.

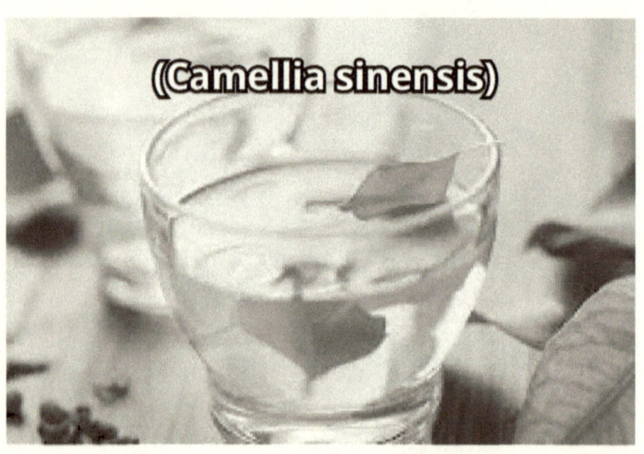

Application:

- After washing your hair with shampoo, pour the green tea on your hair and scalp.
- Massage gently and leave for a few minutes before rinsing with warm water.
- Use as a final rinse once a week to strengthen hair and stimulate growth.

Banana and Honey Mask:

Preparation:

Mash a ripe banana in a bowl and mix it with 1 tablespoon of honey until you get a smooth paste.

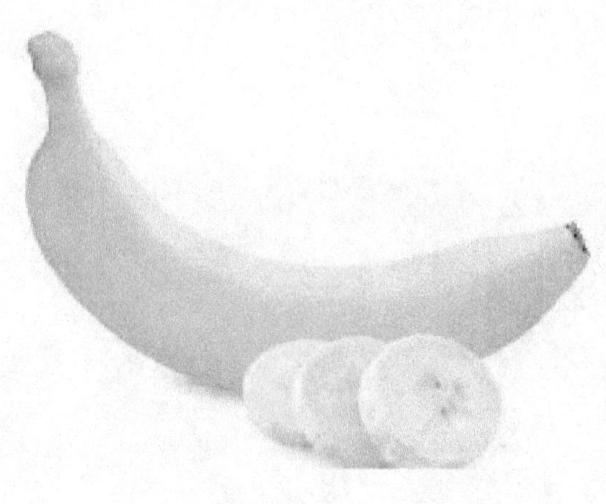

Application:

.Apply the mask to the scalp and hair, covering all areas.
.Leave it on for 30-45 minutes and then rinse with warm water and mild shampoo.
.Use this mask once a week to strengthen hair and reduce hair loss.

Castor Oil (Ricinus communis L.) and Almond Oil (Prunus dulcis):

Preparation:

Mix equal parts castor oil and almond oil in a small jar.

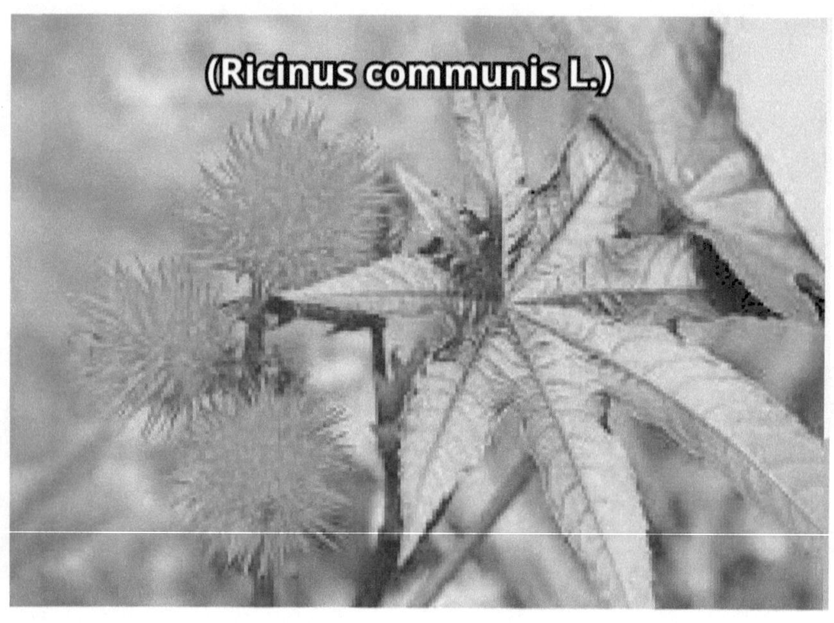

Application:
.Slightly warm the oil mixture and gently massage it into the scalp.
.Leave it on for at least an hour or overnight, then wash your hair with mild shampoo.
.Repeat this treatment 2-3 times a week to strengthen hair and stimulate growth.

Apple Cider Vinegar (Malus domestica) and Mint (Mentha x piperita) Rinse:

Preparation:

.Mix 2 tablespoons of apple cider vinegar with some fresh mint leaves in 2 cups of warm water.

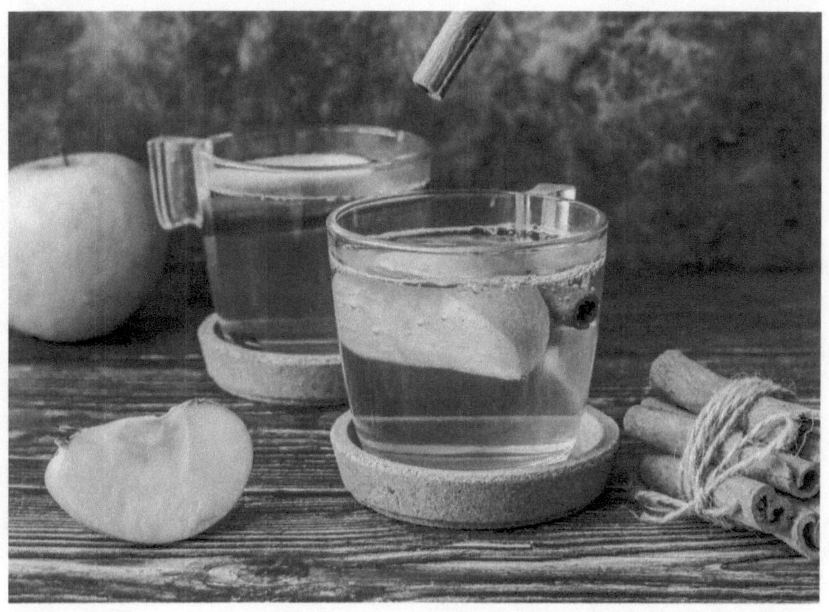

Application:
.After washing your hair with shampoo, pour the apple cider vinegar and mint rinse over your hair and scalp.
.Massage gently and leave for a few minutes before rinsing with warm water.
.Use it as a final rinse once a week to strengthen hair and reduce hair loss.

Papaya (Carica papaya) and Yogurt Mask:

Preparation:

.Mix the pulp of half a ripe papaya with 1/4 cup of natural yogurt in a bowl.

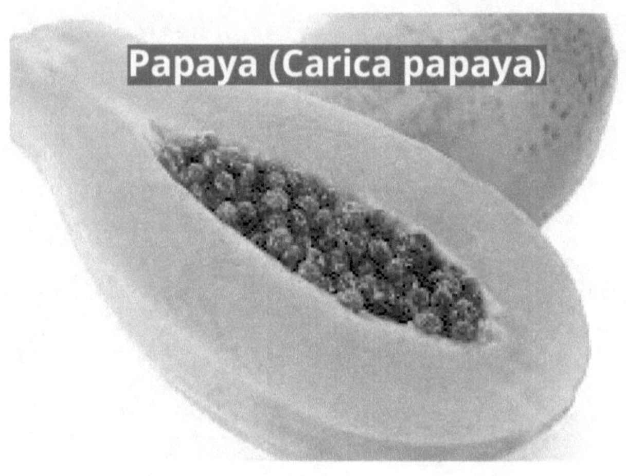

Application:
- Apply the mask to the scalp and hair, covering all areas.
- Leave it on for 30-45 minutes and then rinse with warm water and mild shampoo.
- Use this mask once a week to strengthen hair and reduce hair loss.

Rosemary Tea Infusion:

Preparation:

Boil 2 cups of water and add a few sprigs of fresh rosemary. Let it boil for 10 minutes and then remove from the heat.

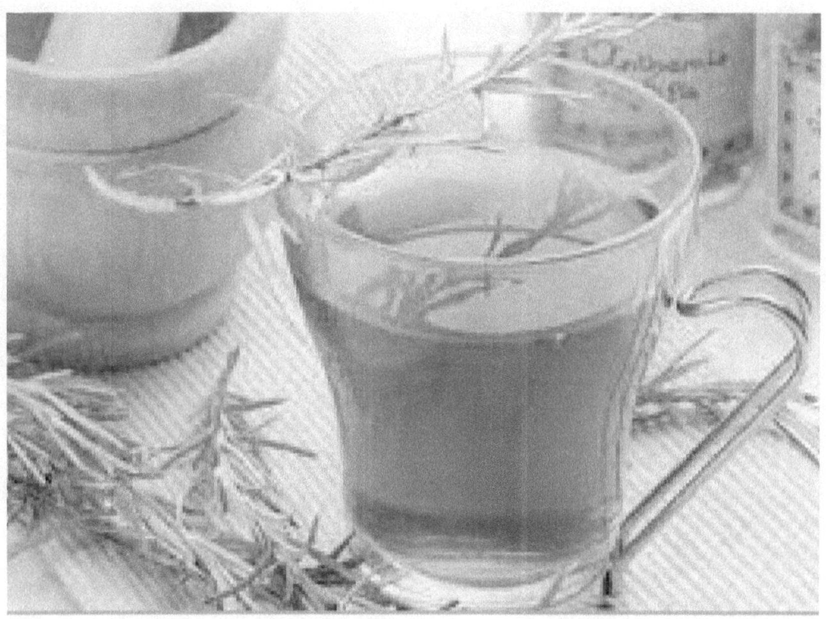

Application:
.Let the rosemary tea infusion cool and then use it as a final rinse after shampooing.
.Massage gently into the scalp and no need to rinse.
.Use this infusion once a week to strengthen hair and stimulate growth.

Turmeric (Curcuma longa) and Coconut Oil (Cocos nucifera) Mask:

Preparation:

.Mix 1 tablespoon of turmeric powder with 2 tablespoons of coconut oil in a bowl.

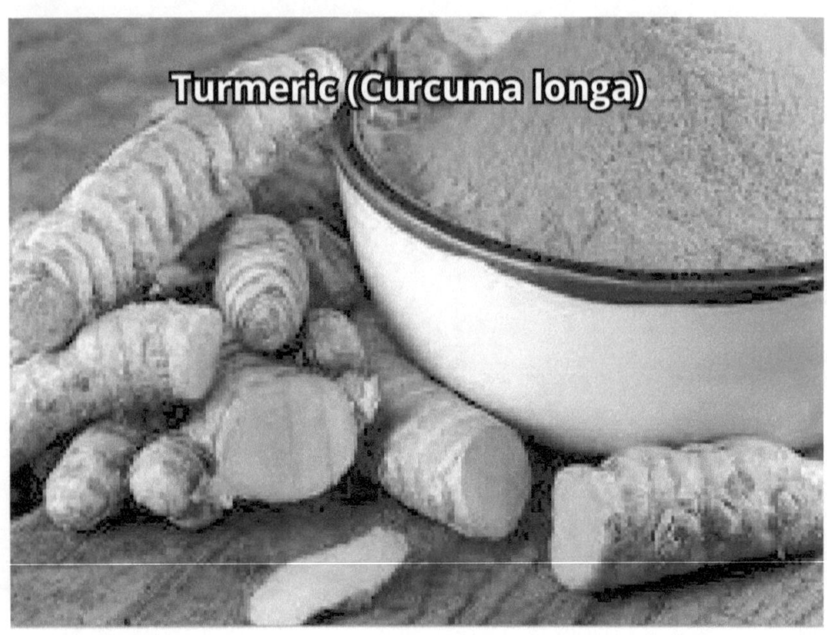

Application:

.Apply the mask to your scalp and hair, making sure to cover all areas.
.Leave it on for 30-45 minutes and then rinse with warm water and mild shampoo.
.Use this mask once a week to strengthen hair and reduce hair loss.

Ginger Tonic (Zingiber officinale):

Preparation:

.Boil 2 cups of water and add a peeled and chopped ginger root. Let it boil for 10-15 minutes, then remove from the heat and let it cool.

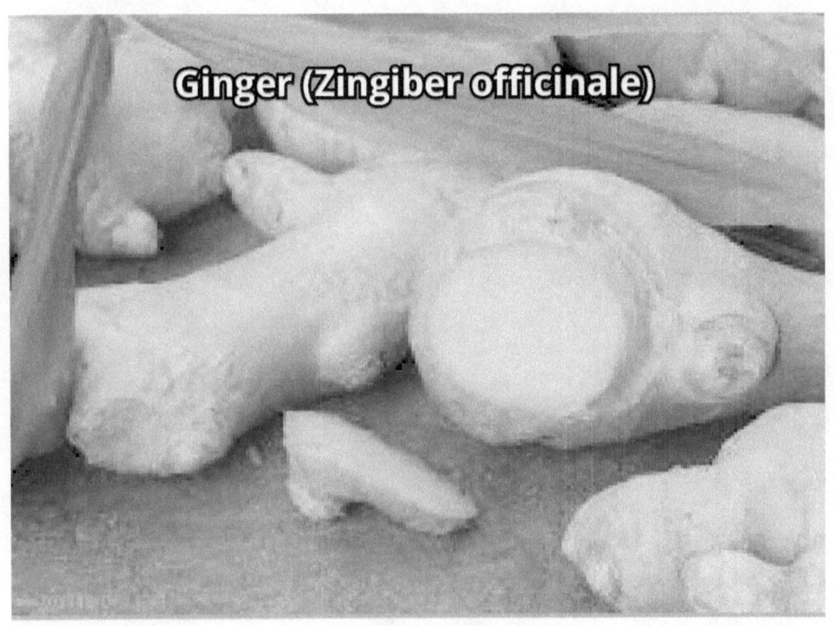

Application:

.Apply the ginger toner to clean scalp and massage gently.
.No need to rinse. Use it as a daily treatment to strengthen hair and stimulate growth

Argan Oil (Argania spinosa) and Egg Mask:

Preparation:

.Mix 1 tablespoon of argan oil with 1 beaten egg in a bowl until you obtain a homogeneous mixture.

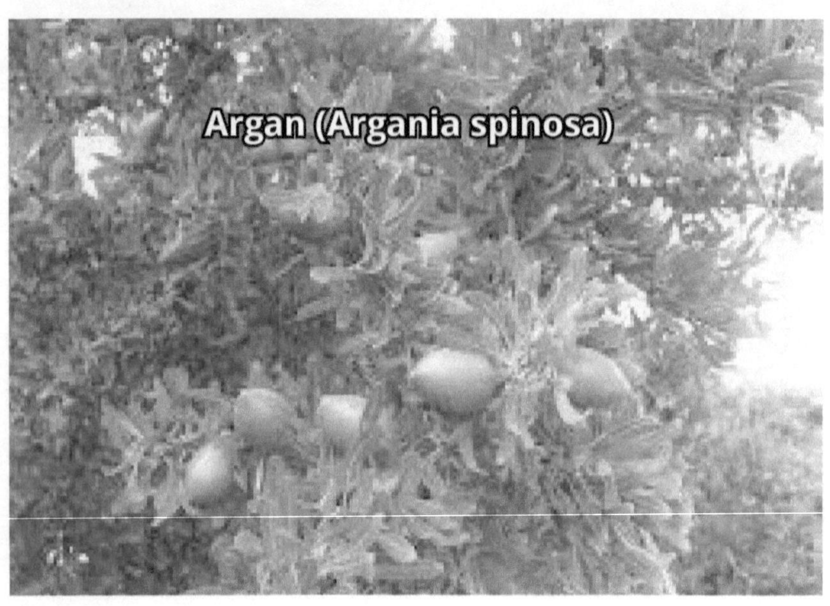

Application:

.Apply the mask to the scalp and hair, covering all areas.
.Leave it on for 30-45 minutes and then rinse with warm water and mild shampoo.
.Use this mask once a week to strengthen hair and reduce hair loss.

These natural treatments offer a variety of options to strengthen and revitalize your hair, reducing hair loss and promoting healthy growth.

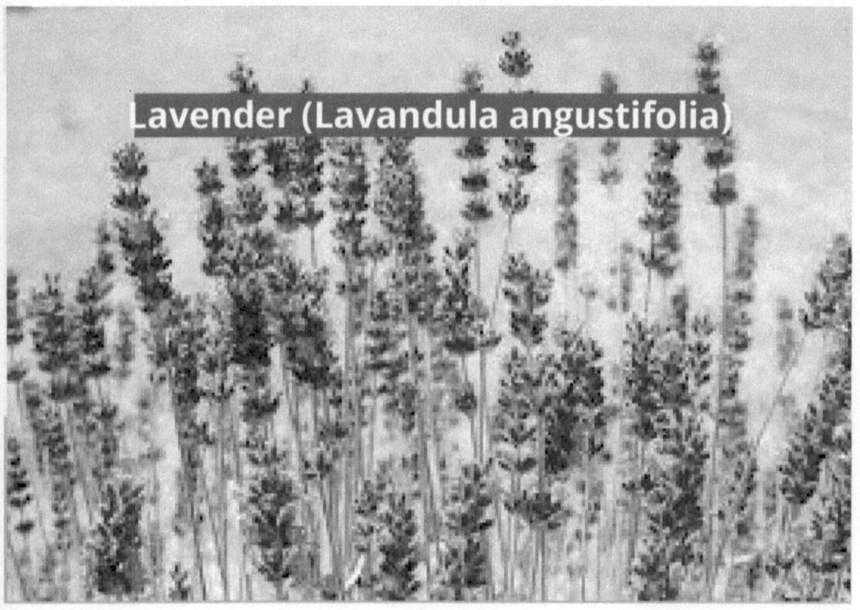

These treatments can help strengthen your hair, reduce hair loss, and promote healthy growth. Remember to be consistent and patient, as the results may take several weeks to become evident.

IV Foods that promote hair care:

1.Avocados (Persea Americana):

They are packed with omega-3 fatty acids, vitamins A, D, and E, as well as protein, which helps strengthen hair, promote growth, and prevent dry scalp.

2.Salmon and Other Fatty Fish: They are rich in omega-3 fatty acids, which are essential for a healthy scalp and shiny hair.

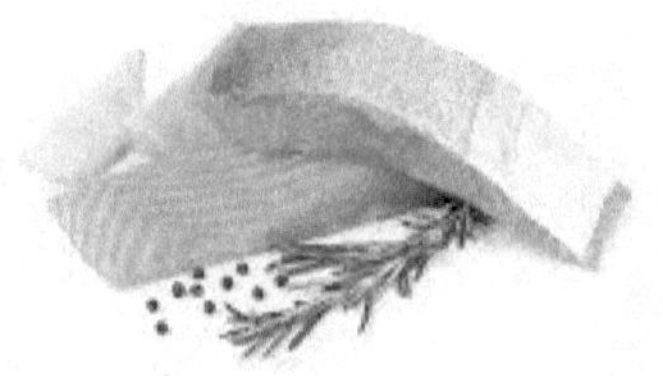

3.Nuts and Seeds:

Almonds, walnuts, sunflower seeds and flax seeds are rich in vitamin E, biotin and fatty acids, which nourish the scalp and promote hair growth.

4.Eggs:

They are an excellent source of protein and biotin, which are essential nutrients for hair growth and the strength of hair follicles.

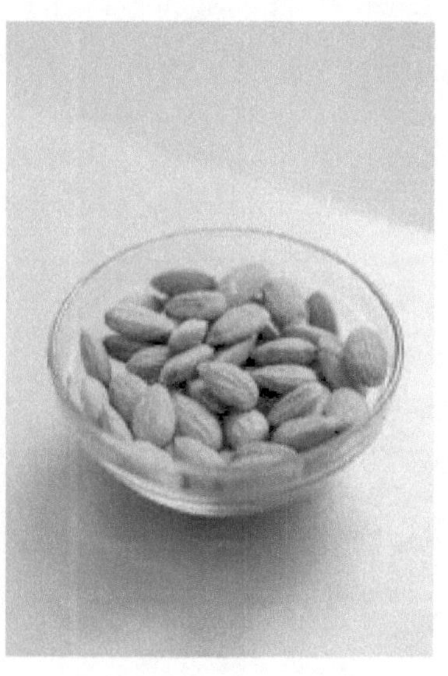

5.Green Leafy Vegetables:

Spinach, kale and chard are rich in iron, vitamin A and vitamin C, which promote sebum production in the scalp and keep hair hydrated.

6.Citrus Fruits:

Lemons, oranges and grapefruits are rich in vitamin C, which helps strengthen hair and promote a healthy scalp.

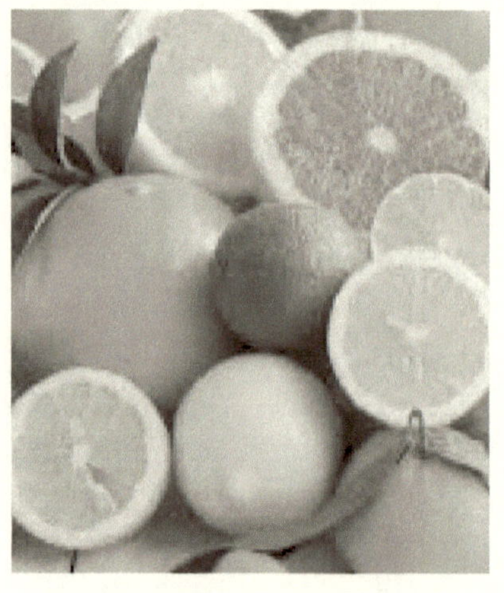

7.Carrots (Daucus carota):

They are rich in vitamin A, which promotes sebum production in the scalp and helps keep hair hydrated and healthy.

8.Potatoes (Ipomoea Potatoes):

They are an excellent source of beta-carotene, which is converted to vitamin A in the body and promotes a healthy scalp and shiny hair.

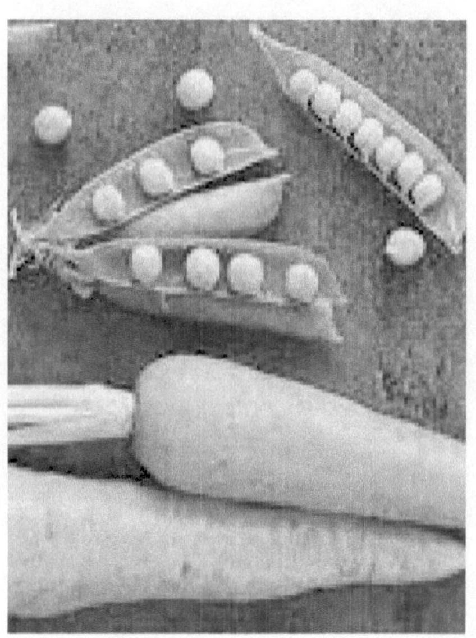

9.Legumes:

Lentils, chickpeas and beans are rich in protein, iron, zinc and biotin, which are essential nutrients for hair health and growth.

10.Dairy products:

Milk, yogurt, and cheese are good sources of calcium, protein, and B vitamins, which are important for hair growth and scalp health.

Incorporating these foods into your daily diet can help strengthen your hair from the inside out, and they can be delicious too!

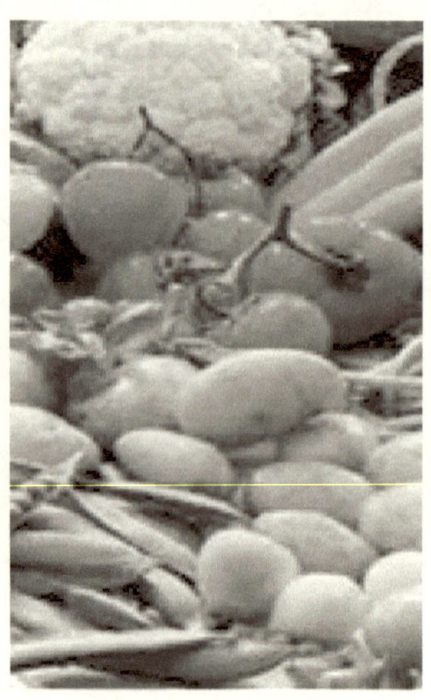

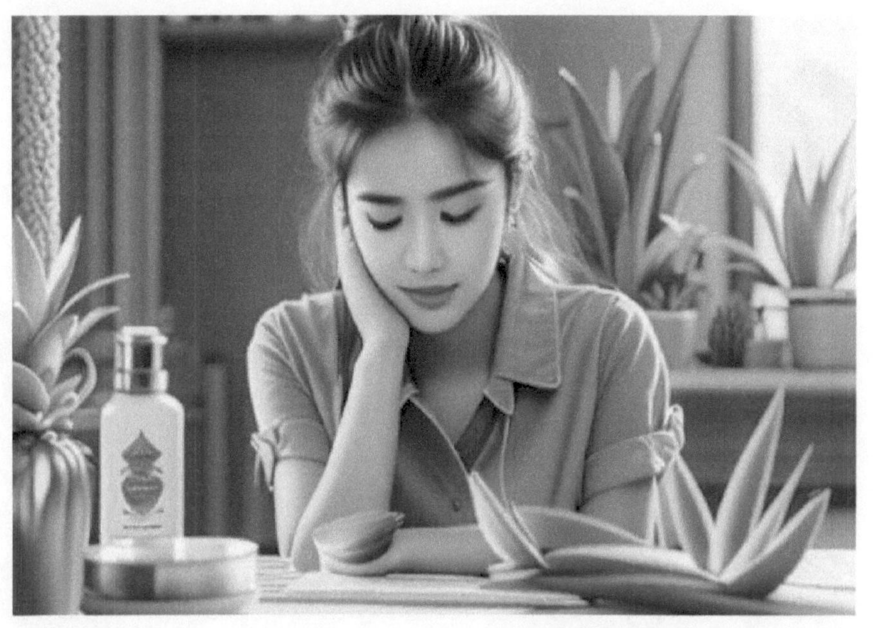

V Expert advice to prevent hair loss

1.Maintain a Balanced Diet: Consuming foods rich in proteins, vitamins and minerals is essential for hair health.
2.Adequate Hydration: Drink enough water to keep your hair and scalp hydrated.

3.Limit Stress: Practice stress management techniques, such as meditation or yoga, to reduce stress levels that can contribute to hair loss.
4.Avoid Tight Hairstyles: Avoid hairstyles that put excessive tension on the hair, such as very tight ponytails or braids.

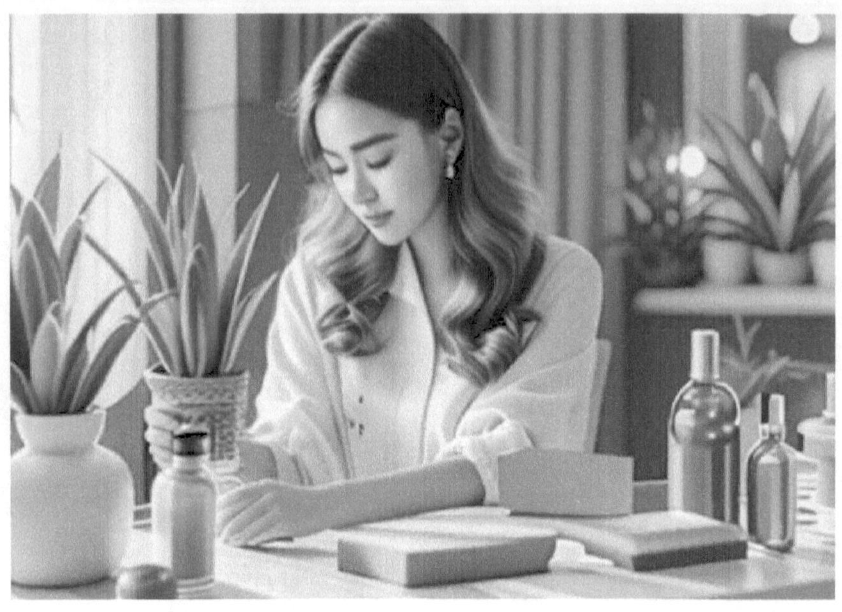

5.Dry your Hair Gently: Avoid rubbing your hair vigorously with a towel when drying it. Instead, dry it gently with a towel or let it air dry.

6.Brush Carefully: Use a soft bristled brush and avoid brushing wet hair, as it is more prone to breakage.

7.Protect your Hair from the Sun: Use hats or products with UV protection to protect your hair from sun damage.

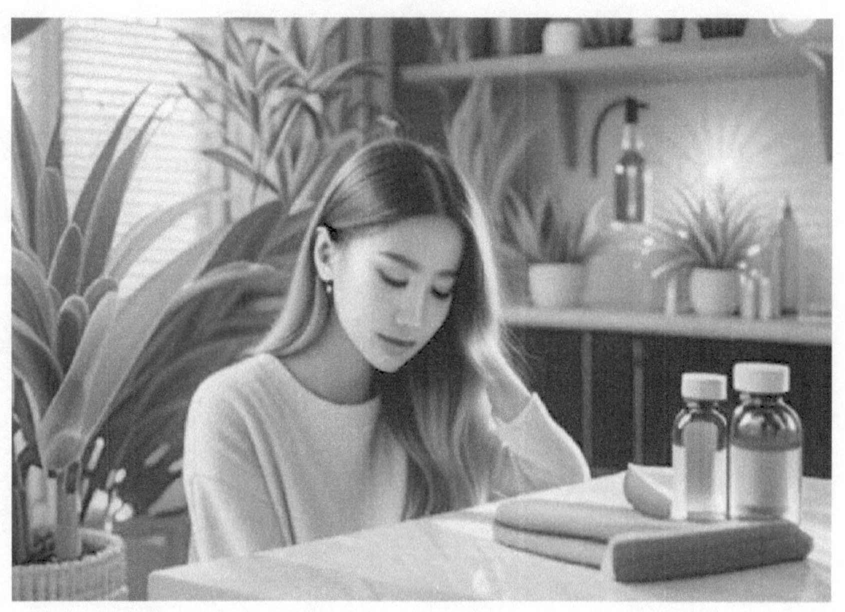

8.Take Care of Your Scalp: Keep your scalp clean and healthy by washing it regularly with a mild shampoo.

9.Avoid Excessive Heat: Limit the use of thermal tools such as hair dryers, straighteners and curling irons, as heat can damage hair.

10.Trim the Ends Regularly: Schedule regular appointments to trim the ends of your hair and prevent splitting and breakage.

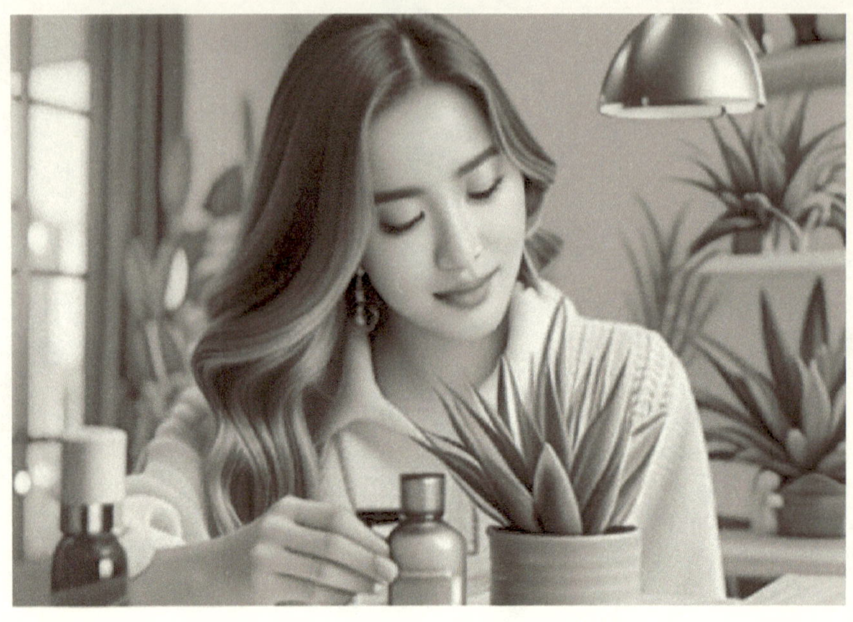

11.Massage your Scalp: Gently massaging the scalp can stimulate blood circulation and promote hair growth.

12.Consume Foods Rich in Biotin: Biotin is an important nutrient for hair health. Find it in foods like eggs, nuts and avocados.

13.Avoid Tobacco: Smoking can affect blood circulation in the scalp and contribute to hair loss.

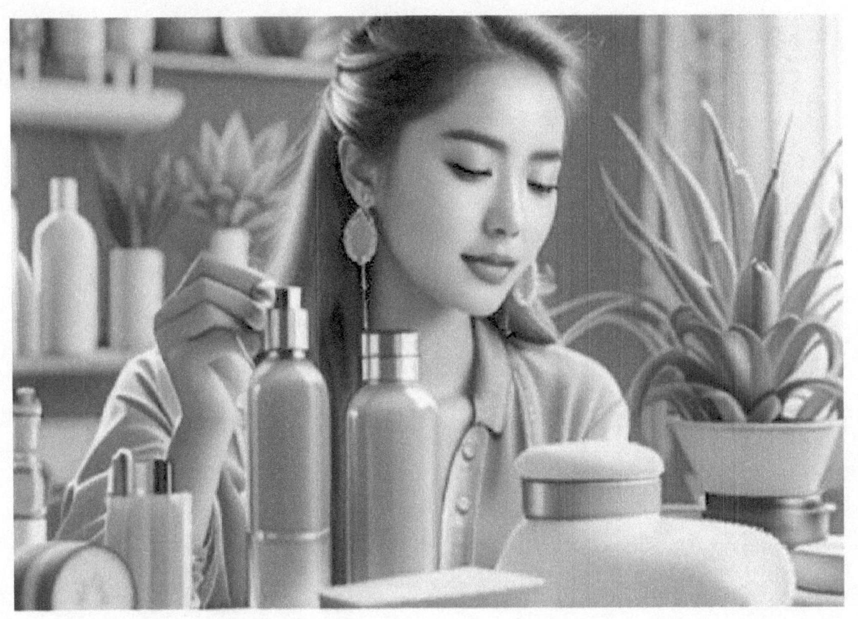

14.Get Enough Rest: Get enough sleep to allow your body to repair and regenerate, which includes hair growth.

15.Consult a Professional: If you experience significant or sudden hair loss, consult a dermatologist or other health professional.

16.Maintain a Healthy Weight: Being overweight and obese can be associated with health problems that can contribute to hair loss.

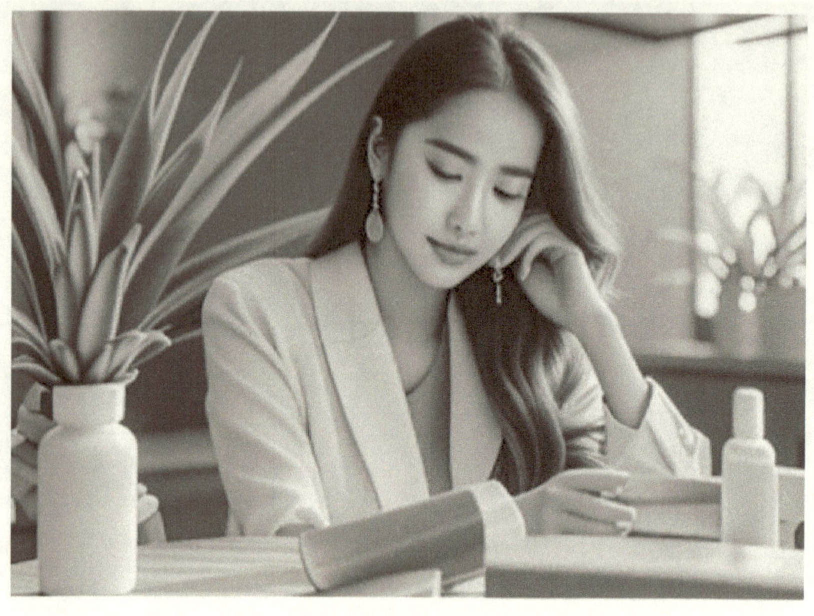

17.Don't Wash Your Hair Too Much: Washing your hair every day can strip the scalp of natural oils, which can cause dryness and damage.

18.Use Gentle Products: Choose mild shampoos and conditioners free of sulfates and parabens to avoid irritation and damage to the scalp.

19.Avoid Excess Chemical Products: Reduce the use of dyes, bleaches and other aggressive chemicals that can damage the hair and scalp.

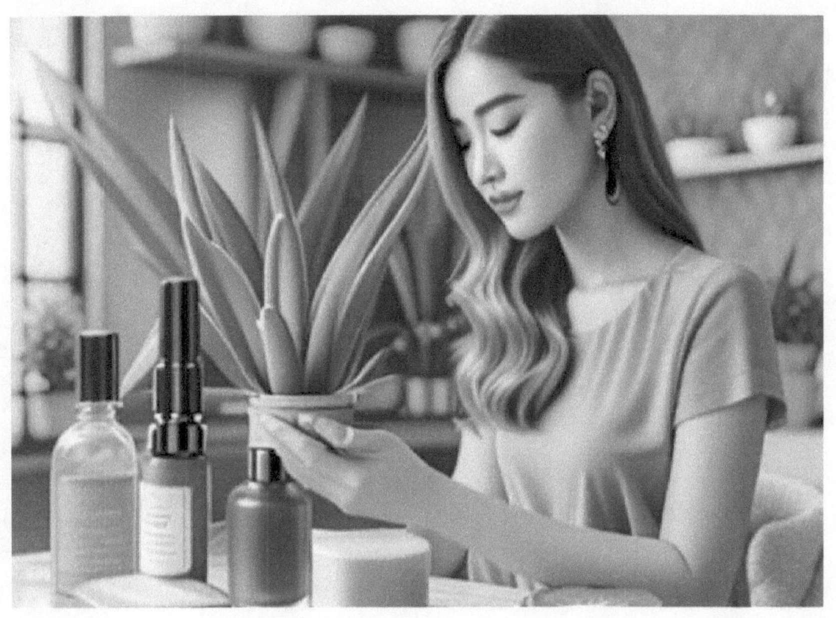

20.Try Natural Treatments: Experiment with natural treatments such as essential oils, clay masks and apple cider vinegar to strengthen and nourish your hair.

21.Supplement with Vitamins and Minerals: Consider taking biotin, vitamin D, iron and zinc supplements if you are not getting enough nutrients from your diet.

22.Avoid Alcohol and Excess Caffeine: Excessive consumption of alcohol and caffeine can dehydrate the body and affect the health of the hair.

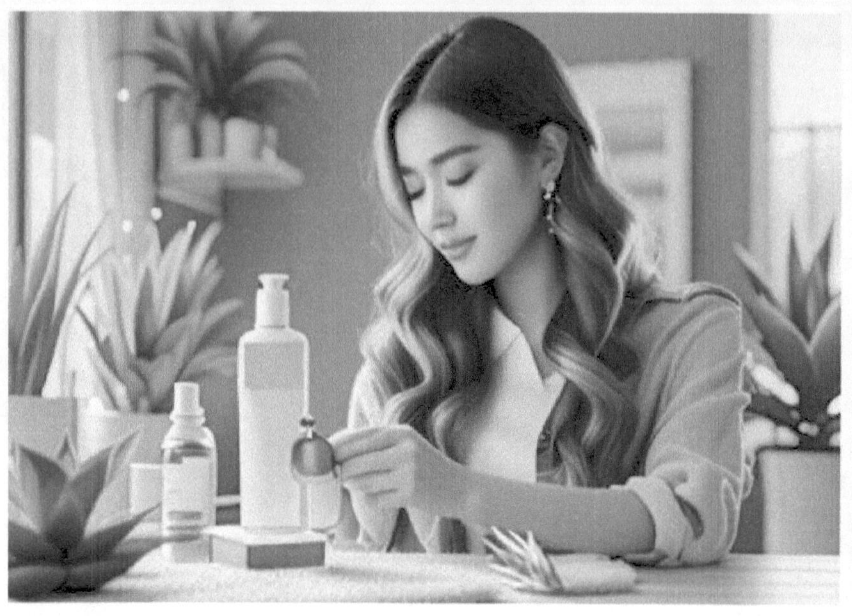

23. Protect your Hair when Swimming: Wear a swimming cap to protect your hair from chlorine and salt in the water.

24.Avoid Smoking: Smoking can contribute to poor blood circulation, which can affect scalp health and hair growth.

25.Control Chronic Diseases: If you suffer from chronic diseases such as diabetes or thyroid, make sure you control them properly, as they may be related to hair loss.

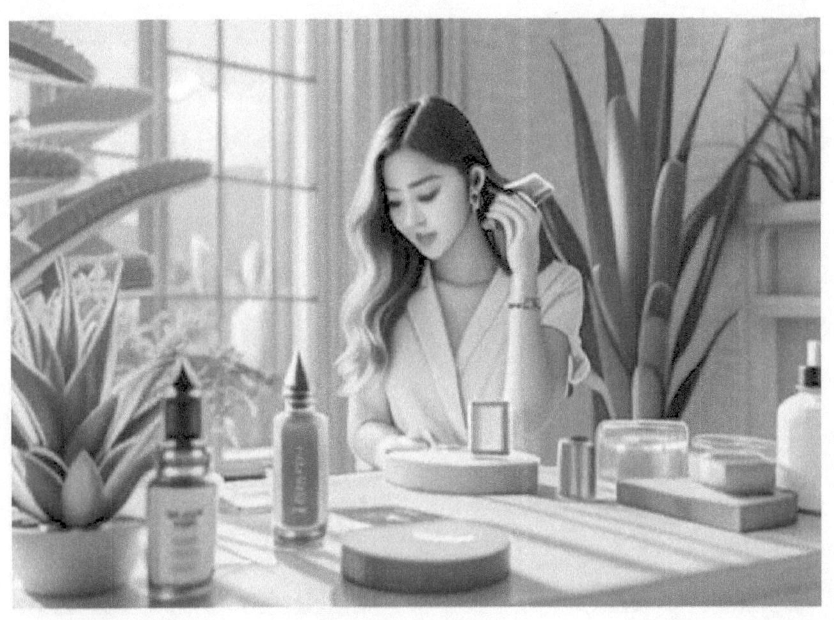

26.Avoid Excessive Manipulation: Avoid excessively twisting, pulling or stretching your hair, as this can weaken it and cause damage.

27.Protect your Hair from the Cold: Wear hats or scarves to protect your hair from the cold and dry wind that can damage it.

28.Maintain Hormonal Balance: If you experience hormonal imbalances, consult a doctor to seek treatment options that can help restore hormonal balance and prevent hair loss.

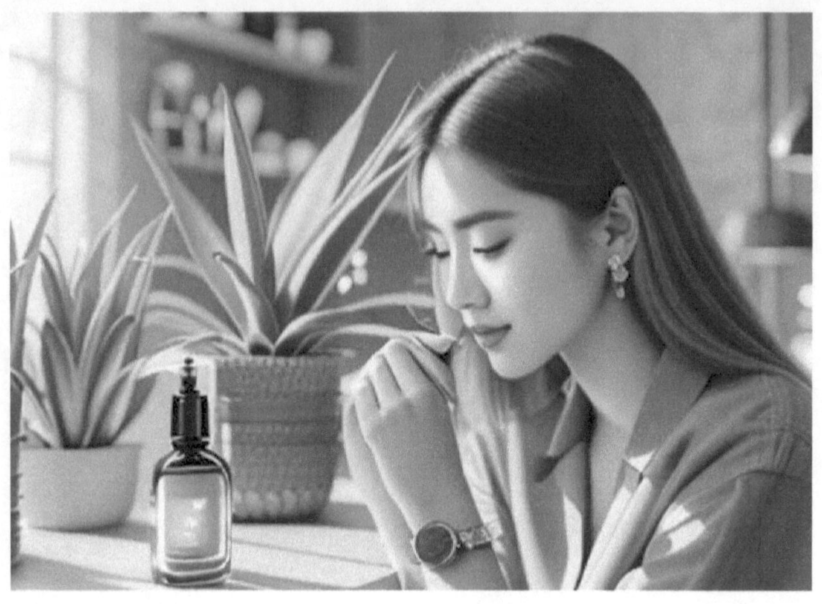

29.Avoid Excessive Stress: Find healthy ways to manage stress, such as exercise, meditation and deep breathing, to reduce its impact on hair health.

30.Consume Omega-3 Fatty Acids: Omega-3 fatty acids, found in foods such as salmon, chia seeds and walnuts, can help strengthen hair and prevent hair loss.

31.Maintain Good Hair Hygiene: Wash your hair regularly to remove oil and dirt buildup that can clog hair follicles and contribute to hair loss.

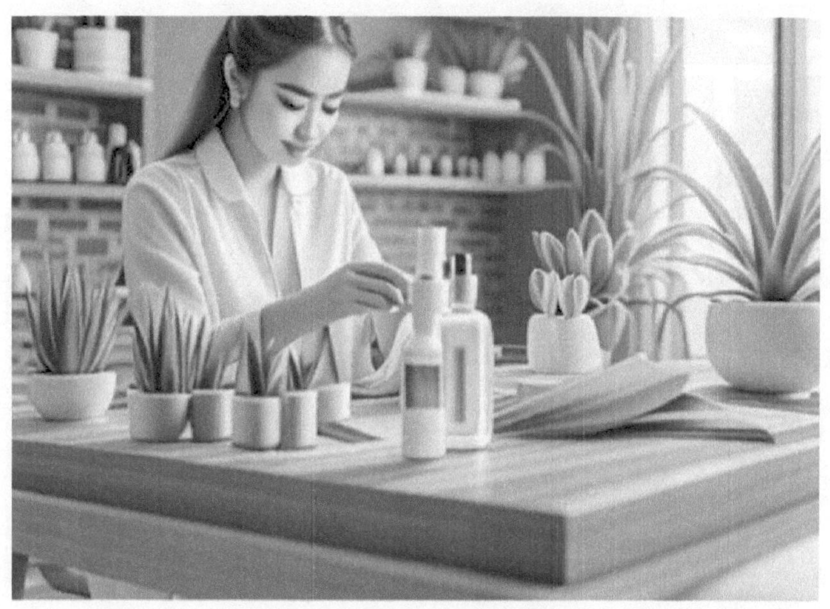

32.Avoid Direct Heat on the Scalp: Avoid exposing your scalp to direct heat, such as intense sun or excessive use of hair dryers, as it can damage the hair and scalp.

33.Avoid Excessive Use of Tight Caps and Hats: Constant use of tight caps and hats can restrict blood circulation to the scalp and contribute to hair loss.

34.Use Hair Treatments in Moderation: Avoid excessive use of hair treatments such as dyes, bleaches and chemical treatments, as they can damage the hair and scalp over time.

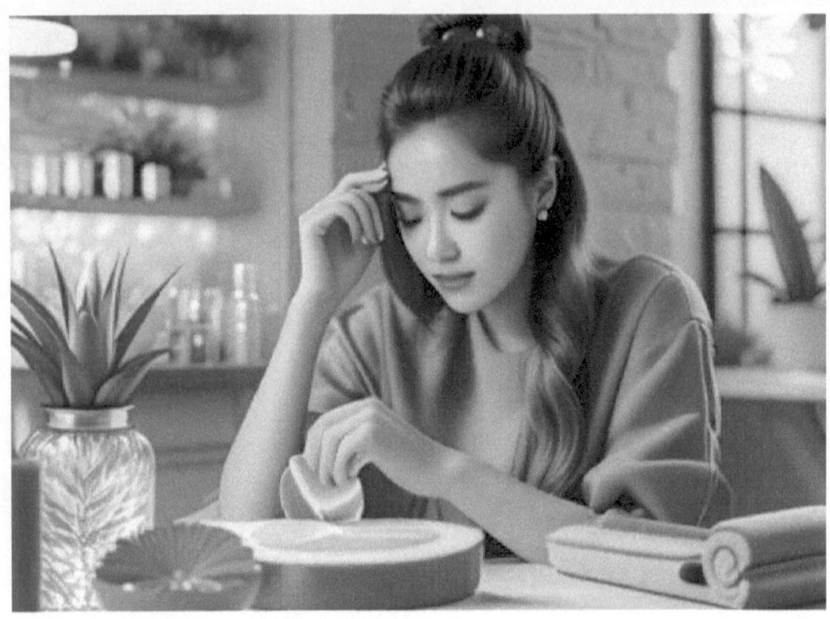

35.Exercise Regularly: Regular exercise can improve blood circulation throughout the body, including the scalp, which can help promote healthy hair growth.

36.Protect your Hair from Chlorine: Before entering the pool, moisten your hair with clean water to reduce the amount of chlorine your hair absorbs.

37.Keep Your Scalp Clean: The buildup of dirt, oil, and hair products on the scalp can clog hair follicles and contribute to hair loss. Wash your hair regularly with a mild shampoo to keep your scalp clean and healthy.

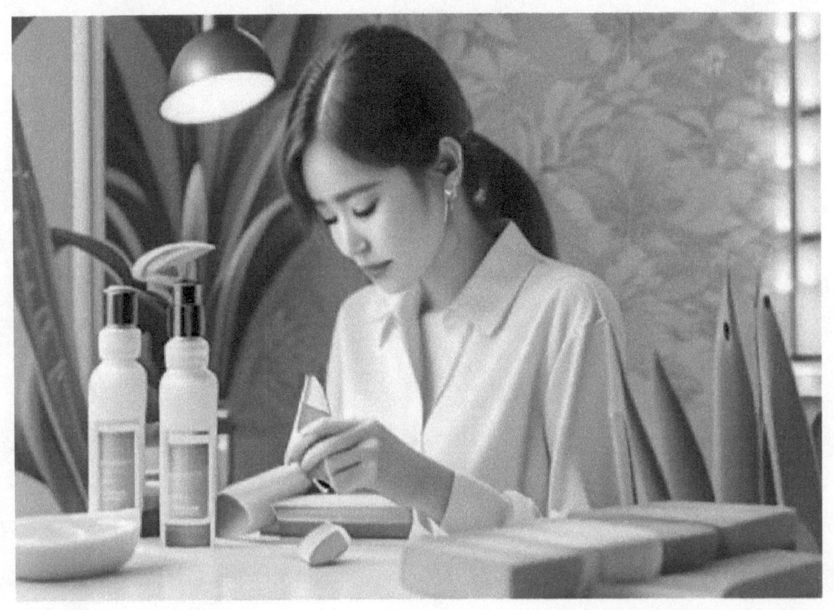

38.Avoid Exposure to Toxic Substances: Exposure to toxic substances in the environment and in personal care products can damage the hair and scalp. Try to avoid exposure to harsh chemicals whenever possible.

39.Have a Regular Checkup: Schedule regular appointments with your dermatologist to check the health of your scalp and hair, especially if you experience significant or sudden hair loss.

40.Be Patient and Consistent: Preventing hair loss requires time, patience and consistency. Don't expect immediate results and continue taking care of your hair with love and dedication.

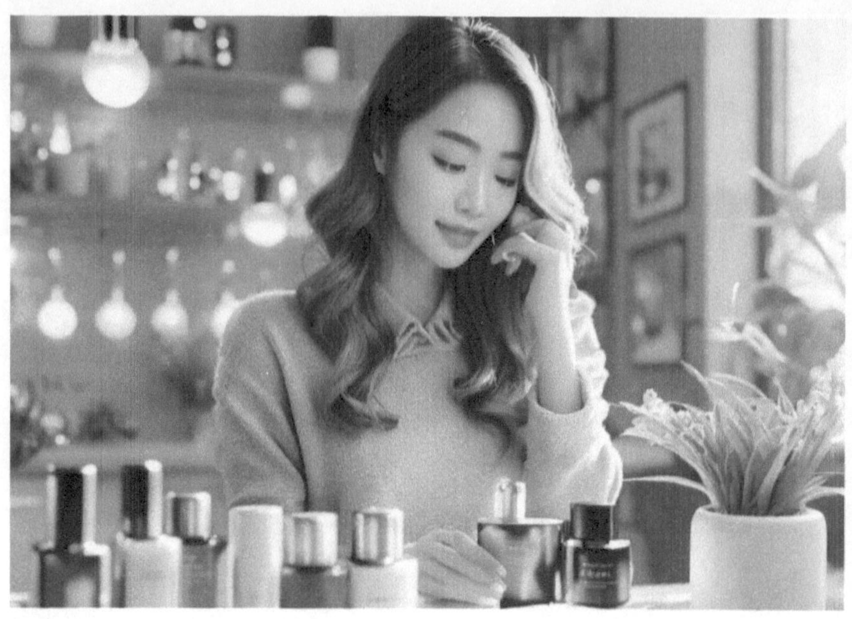

These tips can help you maintain the health of your hair and prevent hair loss.

Remember that each person is unique, so you may need to experiment with different strategies to find the ones that work best for you.

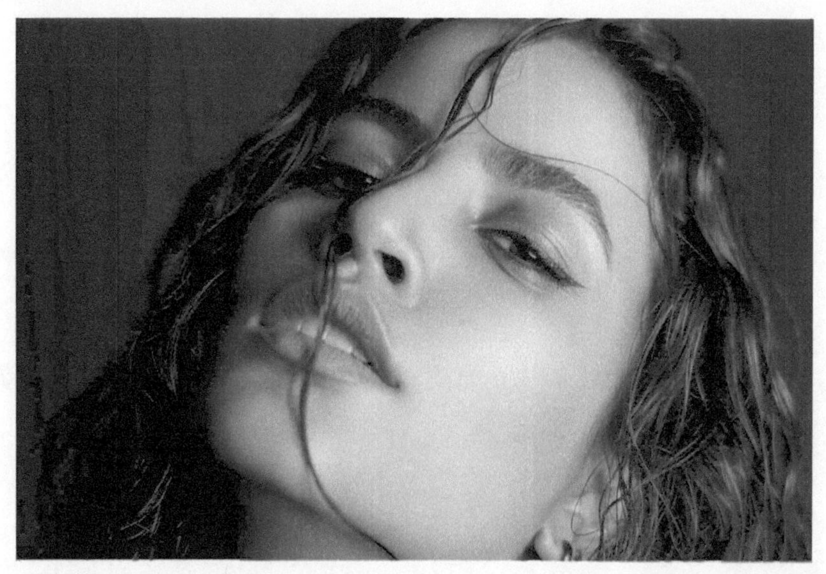

VI Reference to other books of interest

THE ORACLE OF THE FOREST.
https://books2read.com/u/mv66a8

Can´t you sleep?
https://books2read.com/u/bxrqke

Give up alcohol: Learn to live without it
https://books2read.com/u/3yWrMB

You can not sleep?
https://books2read.com/No-puedes-dormir

Road to Sobriety
https://books2read.com/u/49VZ2w

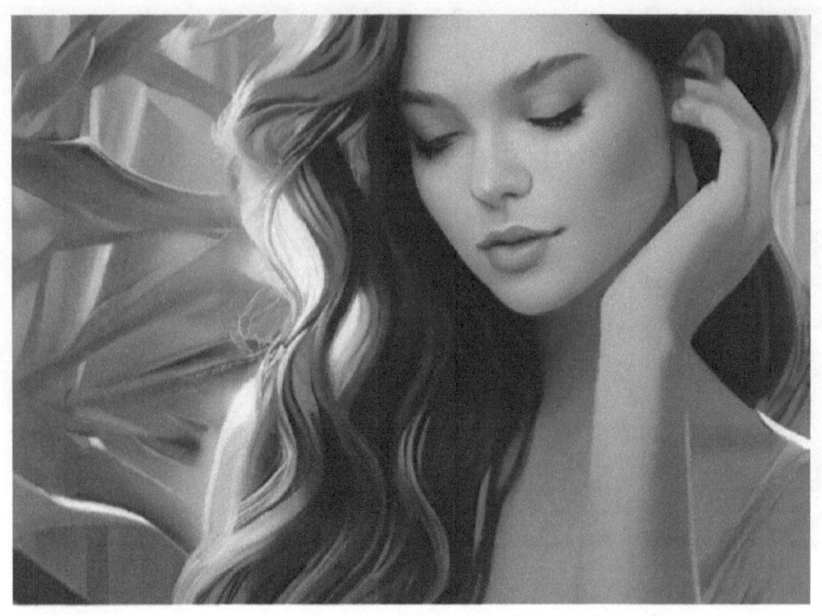

VII Conclusion

In conclusion, hair loss is a common problem that affects people of all ages and genders. Throughout this book, we have explored various causes of hair loss and how natural treatments can be an effective option to restore hair health safely and sustainably.

From homemade masks to herbal teas to dietary changes, we've discovered a wide range of natural approaches that can strengthen hair, stimulate growth, and improve scalp health. These methods not only address the symptoms of hair loss, but also promote overall well-being and a deeper connection with nature.

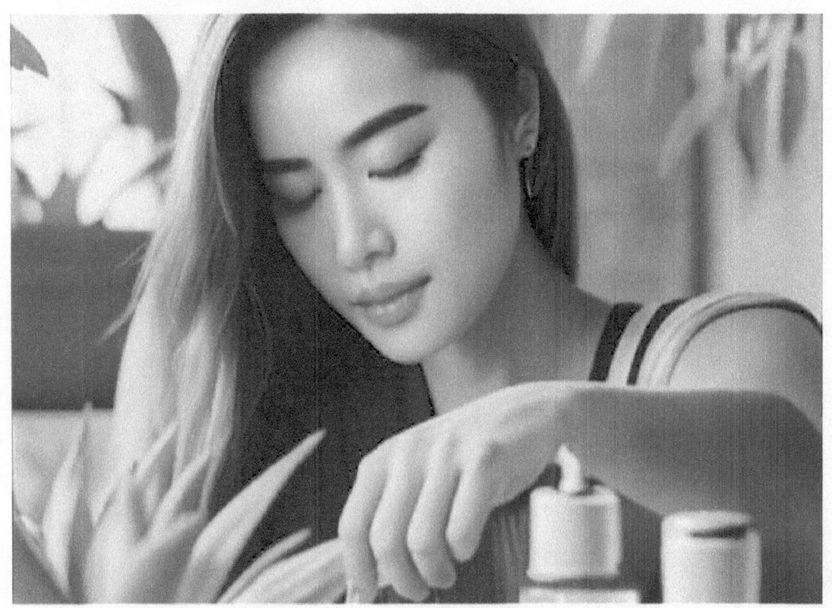

It is important to remember that each individual is unique and may respond differently to treatments. Patience and consistency are key in the hair recovery process. Additionally, it is essential to consult with a health professional if hair loss is persistent or severe, as it may be indicative of underlying conditions that require medical attention.

Ultimately, this book seeks to empower readers with knowledge and tools to address hair loss holistically and naturally. By adopting a comprehensive approach that combines healthy lifestyle habits, body care and natural remedies, we can cultivate strong, radiant and bouncy hair. May this book serve as a guide on your journey toward healthy, beautiful hair, in harmony with nature and with yourself.

VIII ANNEX

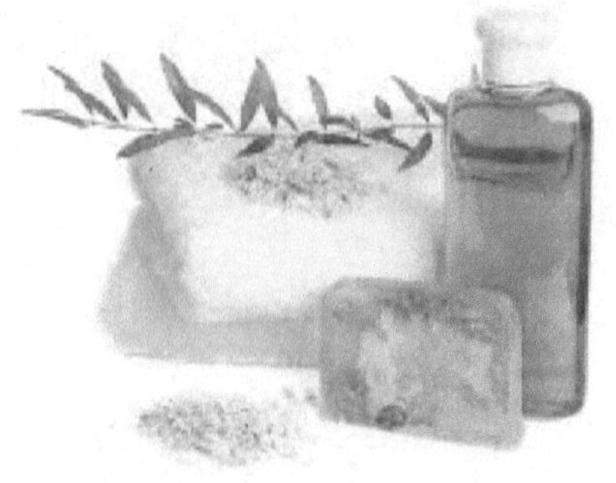

1 Guide to making soap

Recipe to make 20 pieces of handmade soap for hair care

Ingredients:

1.Base oils:

·700 grams of coconut oil ·500 grams of olive oil ·300 grams of sweet almond oil

2.Soda lye (sodium hydroxide):

·270 grams

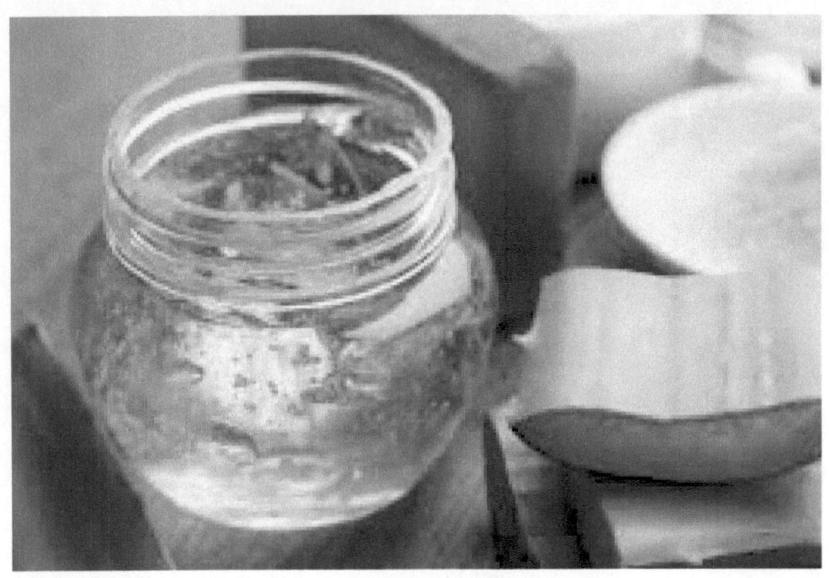

3.Liquid:

·620 grams of distilled water

4.Essential oils:

·20-30 grams in total, depending on the desired fragrance intensity.
·For example, you can use 10 grams of lavender essential oil and 10 grams of rosemary essential oil.

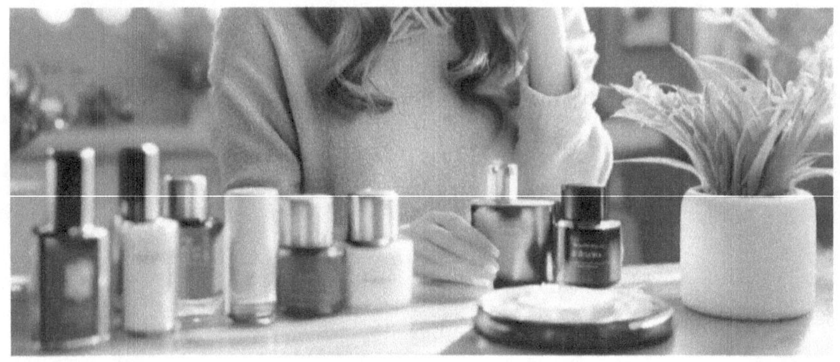

Equipment and process:

1.Security:

·Be prepared with rubber gloves and protective glasses before starting.

2.Measuring ingredients:

·Carefully weigh each of the ingredients.

3. Preparation of the bleach:

·Pour the 270 grams of soda lye into a heat-resistant glass container.
·Add the 620 grams of distilled water to the container with the lye, mixing carefully. Let it cool.

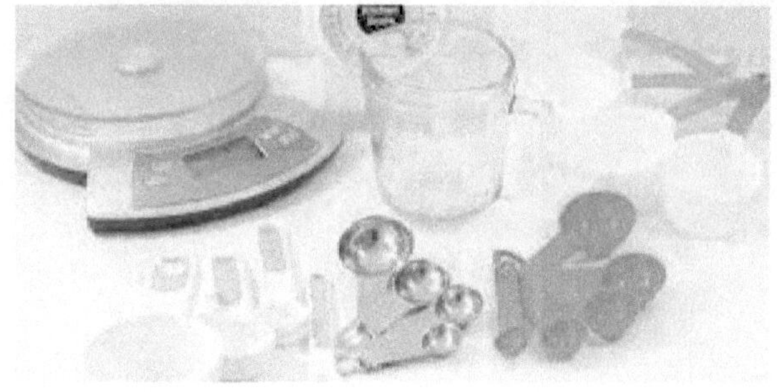

4.Mixture of oils:

·In a heat-resistant container, combine the 700 grams of coconut oil, 500 grams of olive oil and 300 grams of sweet almond oil.
·Heat the oil mixture at a temperature of around 50-60°C until it melts completely.

5.Bleach and oil mixture:

·Once the lye and oils are at the same temperature (around 50-60°C), slowly pour the lye into the oils while constantly mixing with the hand mixer.
·Continue mixing until the mixture reaches the "trace".

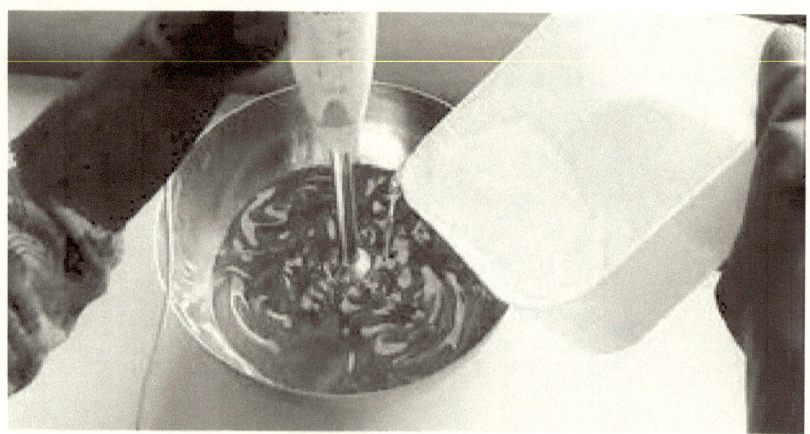

6.Addition of essential oils:

·When the mixture has reached the trace, add the essential oils and mix well.

7 .Pouring into molds:

·Pour the soap mixture into the prepared molds.

8. Soap curing:

·Let the soap sit in the molds for at least 24-48 hours.
·Unmold the soap and cut it into bars of the desired size.

9 .Additional cure:

·Place the soap bars in a cool, dry place to cure for 4-6 weeks.

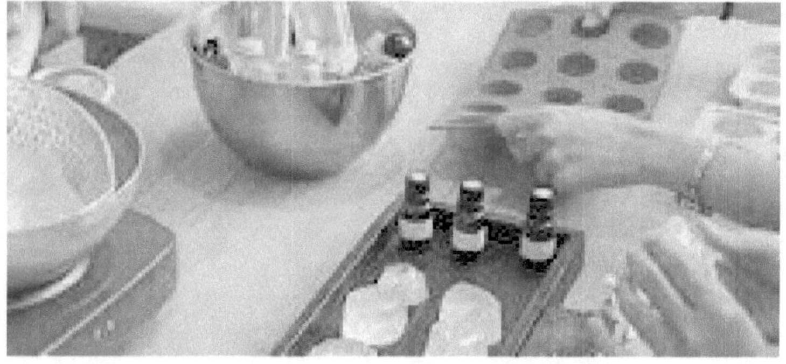

By following this process, you will obtain 20 pieces of natural handmade soap that will be gentle and beneficial for hair care.
Remember to customize the essential oils to your fragrance preferences and enjoy the process of making your own soap.

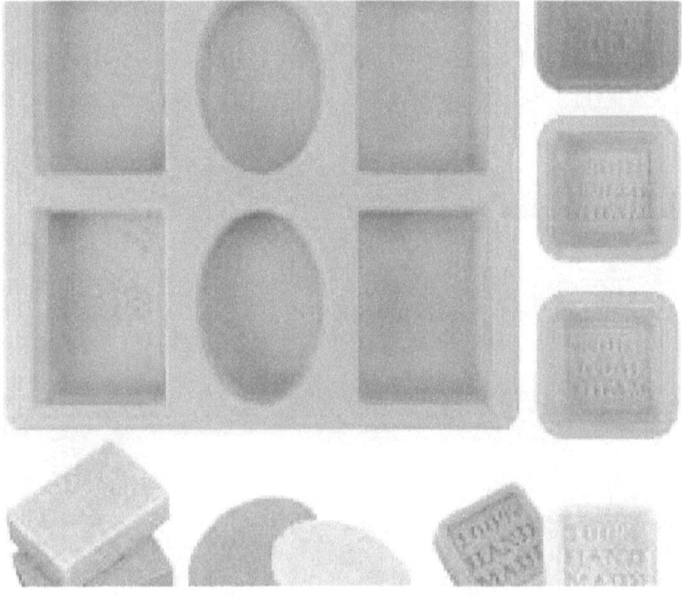

2 Guide to making shampoo

Guide to making shampoo with natural ingredients

This shampoo can help treat hair loss. This recipe focuses on gentle, beneficial ingredients for the scalp and hair:

Ingredients:

1. Distilled water: 500 ml
2. Liquid castile soap: 250 ml
3. Jojoba oil: 30 ml
4. Rosemary essential oil: 10-15 drops
5. Lavender essential oil: 10-15 drops
6. Tea tree essential oil: 5-10 drops
7. Vitamin E (optional): 1 capsule

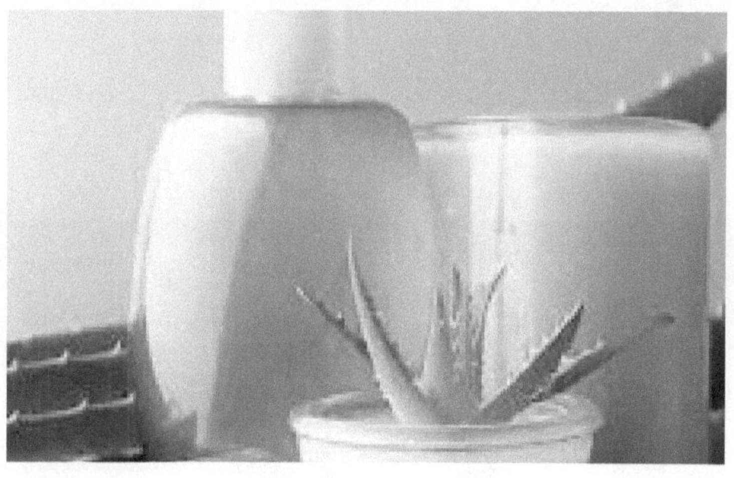

Elaboration process:

1.Mixing liquid ingredients:

·In a large container, pour 500 ml of distilled water.
·Add the 250 ml of liquid castile soap and mix gently to combine.
·

2.Addition of essential oils and vitamin E:
·Add the jojoba oil to the container.
·Squeeze the contents of a vitamin E capsule (if using) into the mixture.
·Add 10-15 drops of rosemary essential oil, 10-15 drops of lavender essential oil and 5-10 drops of tea tree essential oil.
·Mix all the ingredients well to make sure they are completely incorporated.

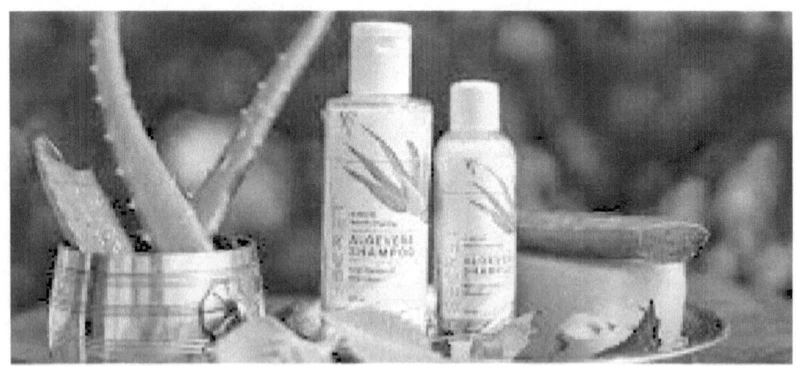

1.Storage and use:

·Pour the shampoo into a glass or dark plastic bottle to protect the essential oils from light.
·Shake gently before use.
·Apply an appropriate amount of shampoo to wet hair and gently massage the scalp.
·Rinse thoroughly with warm water.

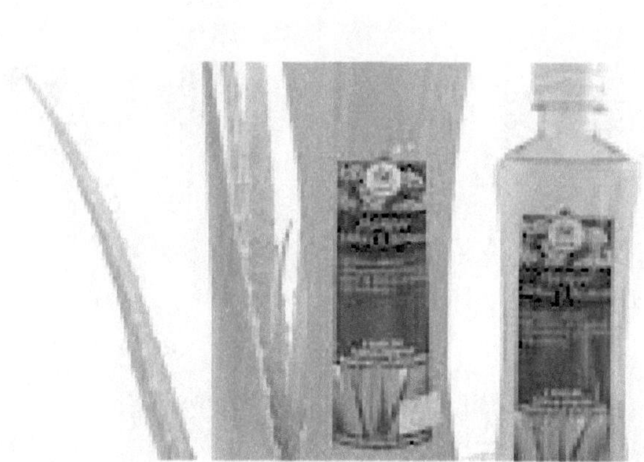

Ingredient benefits:

1.Liquid Castile Soap: It is gentle and contains no harsh chemical ingredients, making it ideal for cleansing hair and scalp without causing irritation.

2.Jojoba oil: Nourishes and moisturizes the scalp, helping to keep hair strong and healthy.

3.Rosemary essential oil: Stimulates blood circulation in the scalp, promoting hair growth and preventing hair loss.

4.Lavender essential oil: It has calming properties that can help reduce inflammation and improve scalp health.

5.Tea tree essential oil: It has antibacterial and antifungal properties that can help keep the scalp clean and free of infections.

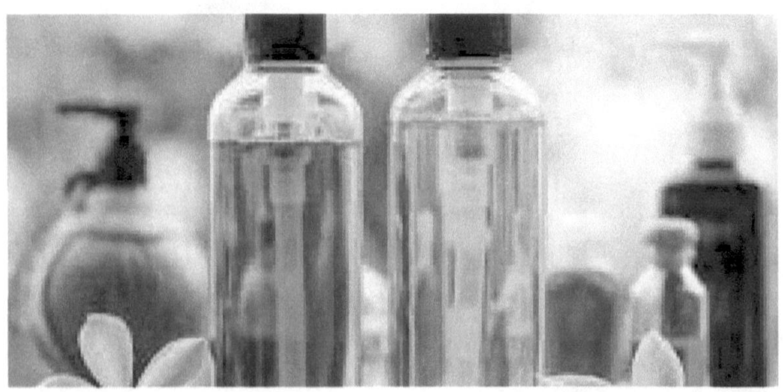

This natural shampoo recipe can be a gentle and effective option to treat hair loss, providing nutrients and stimulating the scalp naturally.

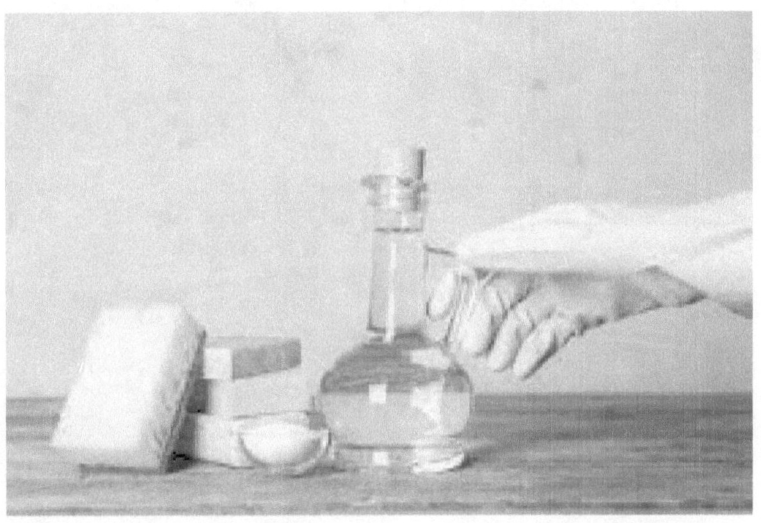

Thank you for having read my book! I hope everything I teach helps you and you put the advice and recommendations into practice. I also hope you give me some stars and a good comment as positive reviews so that more people can read this book.
 See you soon!